NICK MITCHELL & JONATHAN

U.P. ENCYCLOPAEDI
PERSONAL TRAINI

VOLUME 2

BODY TRANSFORMATION
MEAL PLAN DESIGN

HOW TO CREATE DIETS FOR
THE FASTEST POSSIBLE BODY COMPOSITION
IMPROVEMENTS IN MEN AND WOMEN

CONTENTS

INTRODUCTION

**FOREWORD
BY NICK MITCHELL**   6

Success Stories   10

How to Use This Book   12

SETTING UP FOR SUCCESS

Establish Your Starting Point   16

Transformation Time Frames   17

Scheduling Your Transformation   18

Transformation Training   22

• Resistance Training   22

• NEAT   23

• Formal Cardio   26

TRANSFORMATION NUMBERS

How to Calculate Your Nutrition Targets   30

Step 1: Estimate Maintenance   31

Step 2: Set Calorie Target   37

Step 3: Set Macronutrient Targets   39

Transformation Number Case Studies   44

TRANSFORMATION FOODS

Key Points   48

Protein   50

Fat   53

Carbohydrate   56

Drinks and Condiments   59

TRANSFORMATION MEAL PLANNING

Meal Planning Essentials   62

Serving Size FAQs   64

How to Write a Meal Plan   69

Adapting the Meal Plan: Dining Out   75

Adapting the Meal Plan: Refeeds   79

Adapting the Meal Plan: Calorie Shifting   82

Weekly Meal Planning   84

PROGRESS ASSESSMENT

The Ultimate Performance
Body Composition Assessment   88

• Bodyweight   89

• Circumference Measurement   93

• Progress Pictures   96

• Body Fat Percentage   99

• Adherence   103

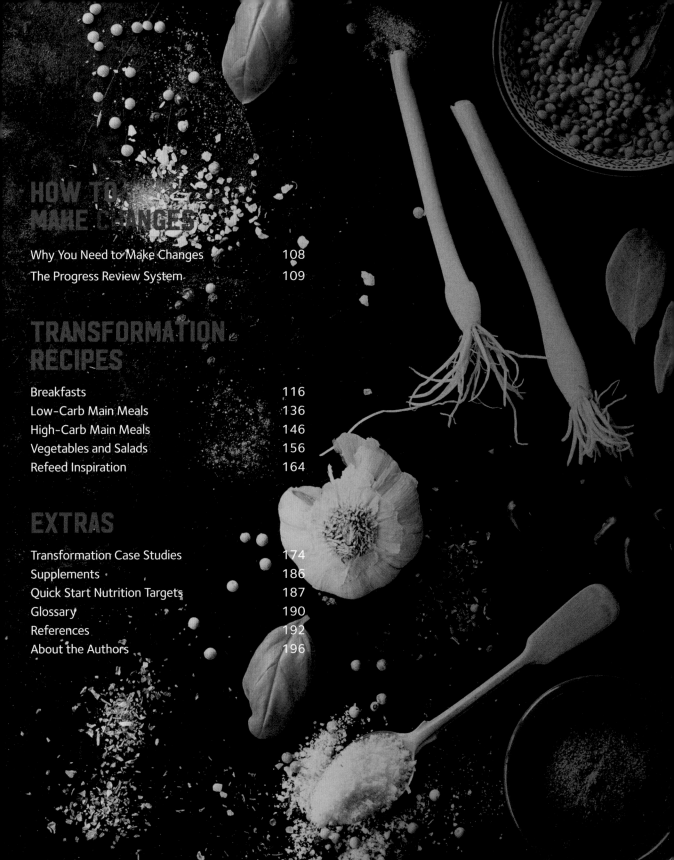

HOW TO MAKE CHANGES

Why You Need to Make Changes   108

The Progress Review System   109

TRANSFORMATION RECIPES

Breakfasts   116

Low-Carb Main Meals   136

High-Carb Main Meals   146

Vegetables and Salads   156

Refeed Inspiration   164

EXTRAS

Transformation Case Studies   174

Supplements   186

Quick Start Nutrition Targets   187

Glossary   190

References   192

About the Authors   196

FOREWORD
NICK MITCHELL

There's a very clear trifecta to body composition success:

- The right exercise regime.
- Optimal stress management.
- The correct diet.

Far and away the most challenging of these factors to get right is the correct diet and yet, perversely, it is also the simplest to establish. Whereas a smart exercise regime takes into account everything from biomechanics to structural balance, and needs to be intelligently planned out in order to maintain ongoing positive adaptations (in other words, progress), and stress management is a veritable minefield of sleep protocols, mental health management and digestive issues, **the actual diet that is optimal for most of us is really rather simple.**

If we aim to "eat from the land" by avoiding Frankenstein foods and sticking to nutrition that we can kill, pick, or pluck, all whilst eating fewer calories than we expend then most of us can get as lean as we want to be. Combine that with the right amount of resistance training and some amazingly wonderful (often unbelievable to some, if you look at U.P.'s results) outcomes can be achieved in startlingly short time frames.

After all the labour that's gone into this book I hesitate to write this, but if most of us ate three meals a day from the "kill it, pick it, pluck it" list with no snacks in between, we'd destroy the obesity epidemic, put personal trainers out of business, and much of this book would be superfluous to your needs.

Life, however, is rarely so simple.

IF WE AIM TO "EAT FROM THE LAND" BY AVOIDING FRANKENSTEIN FOODS AND STICKING TO NUTRITION THAT WE CAN KILL, PICK, OR PLUCK, ALL WHILST EATING FEWER CALORIES THAN WE EXPEND THEN MOST OF US CAN GET AS LEAN AS WE WANT TO BE.

Whilst "knowing" what to eat is so straightforward that it can be bundled into just a few simple rules, the reality of picking a diet that someone can live with and stick to is an entirely more challenging proposition. Almost every second of our waking lives, sophisticated and

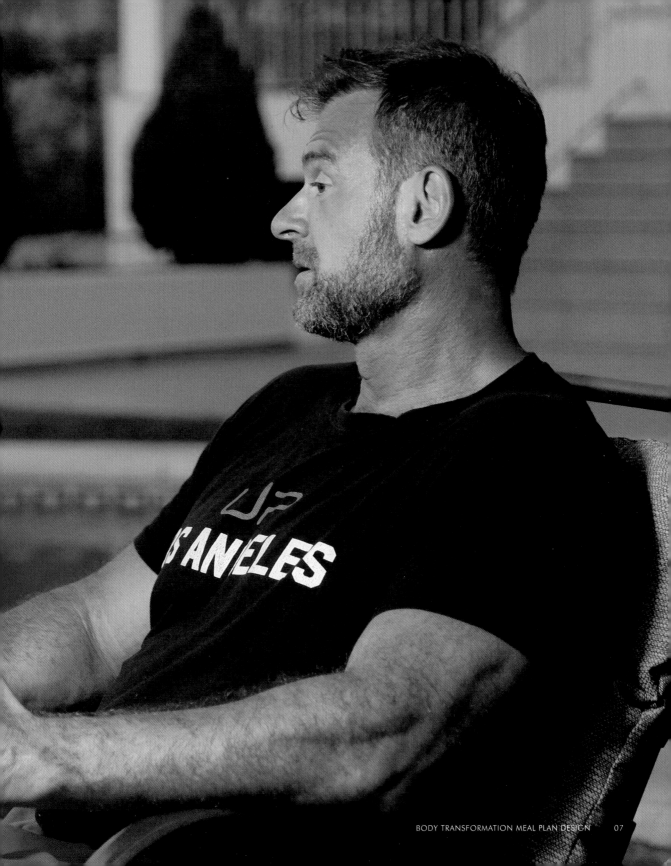

alluring food providers bombard us with temptation to stray off plan. After all the occasional little bit of what I fancy won't hurt me, right?

Yes, that is correct. But how many of us can properly control the size or the frequency of that "fancy"? Not a lot if the frightening and shameful global obesity statistics are any measure.

What we have learned, via over a decade of working one-to-one with tens of thousands of personal training clients are the following rules:

1) There's no such thing as the "perfect diet". Anything being sold to anybody as such is a pure sham and a money-making vehicle.

2) Whereas many approaches to dieting can be effective, there are universal rights and wrongs, such as maintaining the appropriate protein intake and "calories do count".

3) Starvation diets work in the short term if all you care about is dropping weight, but in reality they screw you up in so many ways that aside from the occasional handful of days going very low calorie, in a way that could be compared to intermittent fasting, they are best to be avoided like the plague. You won't get the long term metabolic shutdown that some hucksters purport, but you will crash in the short term a host of very powerful hormones leading to both a physiological and psychological rebound that oftentimes see you end up fatter than when you started!

4) The single golden rule lies in working with yourself or your client to find out the best diet that can be followed. This is such an important point that it bears repetition:

"The most important aspect to effective dieting lies in finding the plan that you can follow"

5) For some people this can be as simple as "ten rules to eat by", but what we have found at U.P. is that the vast majority of successful transformations follow a set plan. That plan can, and does, vary quite significantly from person to person, but nevertheless having a plan is what works best to prevent all the second guesses, self-justifications, and bad decisions that are the universal plague of the dieter and the reason why over 98% of diets fail in the long term.

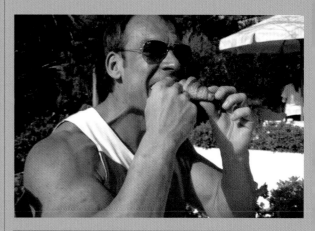

ALMOST EVERY SECOND OF OUR WAKING LIVES, SOPHISTICATED AND ALLURING FOOD PROVIDERS BOMBARD US WITH TEMPTATION TO STRAY OFF PLAN. AFTER ALL THE OCCASIONAL LITTLE BIT OF WHAT I FANCY WON'T HURT ME, RIGHT?

The entire premise of this book is to show you how to construct meal plans that work for you, but don't be fooled into believing that this is a one-size-fits-all meal plan guide. You're going to be required to think a bit, but I make no apologies for that because it's by far the best way to help you achieve your ultimate goal of a leaner, fitter body.

A WORD ON FLEXIBLE DIETING

Somewhere in all the online dieting dogma that confuses even me at times, you'll find the zealots who tell you that "flexible dieting" and its close cousin 'if it fits your macros', more popularly known as IIFYM, are the best ways to eat to get lean.

It's easy for me, someone who doesn't appreciate being fed a line of bullshit, to really oppose the flexible dieting proponents because, in the world of personal training, I know that this advice is wrong for most clients when they're starting out. However, we can't throw the baby out with the bathwater, and long term a flexible dieting approach is very often a wise solution once all the habits, education, and dare I go all broscience and say "metabolic reset" has been locked in place. All of which comes after you've learned how to build meal plans that work!

First some quick definitions:

IIFYM means you can eat what you want so long as it fits your macronutrient targets (protein/fat/ carbohydrate, which we address in *Transformation Numbers*). The problem is that the emphasis is too often placed on hitting those targets irrespective of nutritional quality.

Can IIFYM work if we adhere to sound nutritional practices that are as simple as choosing the right foods? Absolutely. However, too many people can fall into the trap of thinking that if they're getting their carbs and fat from chocolate bars, then they're doing the right thing. We all know this isn't right, but when it comes to dieting with most people, especially when they're starting out, give them an inch, and they take a mile.

The exact same principles hold true for the concept of flexible dieting. Put simply, this is a less strict, more user-friendly version of IIFYM and one that should ultimately form the bedrock of most people's eating habits. I'm firmly of the view that most of us don't want to be chained to spreadsheets and number counting when enjoying our meals.

Flexible dieting in my world is simple common sense eating. It means keeping an eye on a few numbers, at bare minimum we want to have an idea of a daily protein goal and rough calories, and to balance out the days that you go overboard you have days that you go under.

The problem with IIFYM and flexible dieting is that the overwhelming majority of us lack the ability to properly control our eating habits which is where the value of the right meal plan always comes in.

Committing to writing and following a meal plan will teach you several eye-opening lessons about how your eating habits affect your body composition.

We also know from our experience working with clients that achieving transformational results in a short time frame requires a disciplined and measured approach.

Once you have achieved your transformation, you can use your newfound dietary awareness to transition to a more flexible and sustainable approach.

FLEXIBLE DIETING IN MY WORLD IS SIMPLE COMMON SENSE EATING. IT MEANS KEEPING AN EYE ON A FEW NUMBERS, AT BARE MINIMUM WE WANT TO HAVE AN IDEA OF A DAILY PROTEIN GOAL AND ROUGH CALORIES, AND TO BALANCE OUT THE DAYS THAT YOU GO OVERBOARD YOU HAVE DAYS THAT YOU GO UNDER.

SUCCESS STORIES

There's a common misconception that rapid results are just a marketing gimmick and can only be "gamed" via photoshop, fake time lines, drugs, or detraining a formerly fit person and then taking advantage of "muscle memory" to get the subject into shape in record time.

Whilst all of this goes on far too much in the wider fitness industry, it doesn't happen at U.P.. Our clients are not aspiring fitness models or bodybuilders, they are regular people who want to maximize the efficiency of their fitness regimes.

Here's a little look at a wide selection of people who have made rapid changes all whilst holding down full-time, often stressful, careers and only coming into the gym three to four times a week. Never let anyone tell you that it can't be done, the power of highly-focused commitment and the right training and diet plan can work wonders!

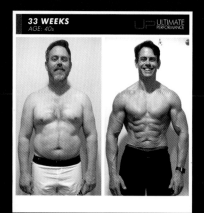
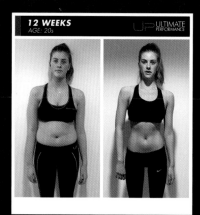
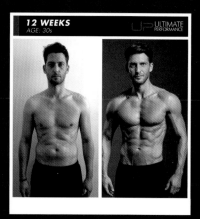

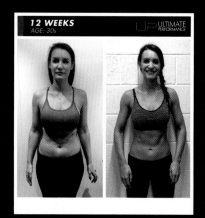
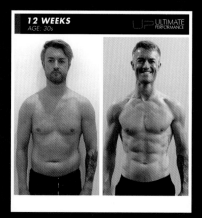
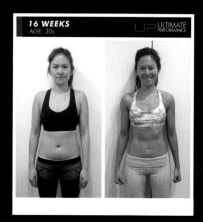

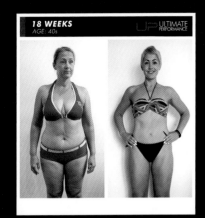

18 WEEKS
AGE: 40s

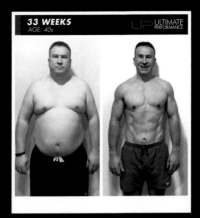

33 WEEKS
AGE: 40s

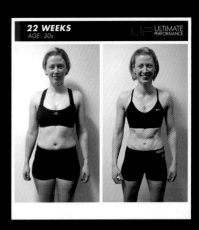

22 WEEKS
AGE: 30s

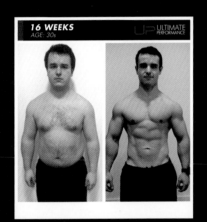

16 WEEKS
AGE: 30s

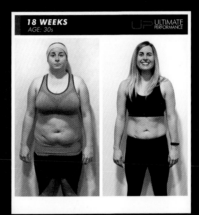

18 WEEKS
AGE: 30s

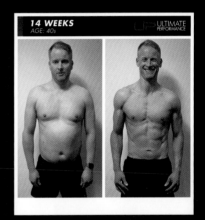

14 WEEKS
AGE: 40s

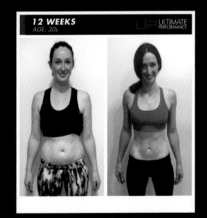

12 WEEKS
AGE: 30s

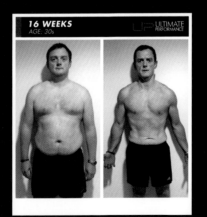

16 WEEKS
AGE: 30s

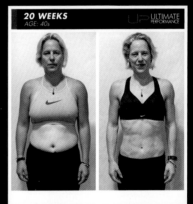

20 WEEKS
AGE: 40s

WILL YOU BE NEXT?

INTRODUCTION
HOW TO USE THIS BOOK

WE HAVE CREATED 'BODY TRANSFORMATION MEAL PLAN DESIGN' BASED ON THE SAME TRANSFORMATION FRAMEWORK THAT WE USE WITH OUR ONE-TO-ONE CLIENTS.

The framework consists of six steps, which we will guide you through below.

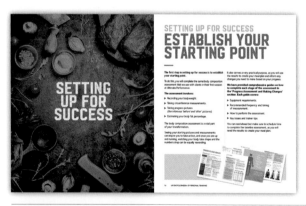

#1 Setting Up for Success

▶ Complete a body composition assessment to establish your starting point and get the information needed to create your meal plan.

▶ Schedule your transformation by selecting your start/end dates and identifying key events that may affect your progress.

▶ Learn about the role of training and regular physical activity in your transformation program.

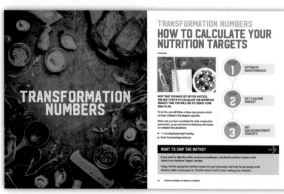

#2 Transformation Numbers

▶ Learn about how many calories and nutrients your body needs (plus the vital roles they perform in your body).

▶ Calculate nutrition targets to build your meal plan around.

▶ If you want to skip the maths, we have provided pre-calculated nutrition targets in the 'Extras' section.

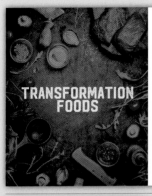

#3 Transformation Foods

▶ All you need to know about the recommended food and drink that you will use to meet your nutrition targets.

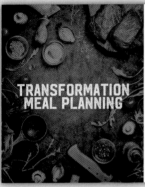

#4 Transformation Meal Planning

▶ This section teaches you basic meal planning skills like how to prepare meals to meet specific nutrition targets.

▶ Follow a step-by-step guide to write your meal plan.

▶ Learn how to adapt your meal plan to stay on track at all times.

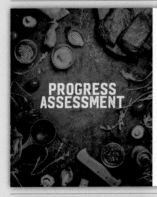
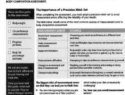

#5 Progress Assessment

▶ Find out how to complete each stage of the Ultimate Performance body composition assessment.

▶ The assessment involves recording your bodyweight, estimating your body fat percentage and taking circumference measurements and progress pictures.

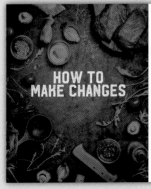

#6 How to Make Changes

▶ Discover the reasons why you might need to make changes to your meal plan during your transformation.

▶ Learn the system we use to interpret our clients' rate of progress and make any required changes to their meal plans.

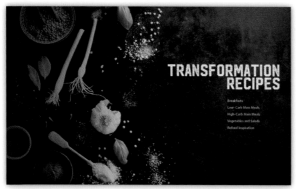

Transformation Recipes

▶ Learn how to combine individual foods into meals that are easy to make, fit with your nutrition targets and that taste delicious!

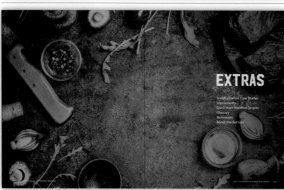

Extras

▶ Case studies: find out how six real-life U.P. clients achieved their outstanding transformations.

▶ Recommended supplement protocol to support your meal plan.

▶ Quick start nutrition targets to fast track your meal plan design.

If you have any questions, do not hesitate to get in touch via one of our social media channels.

We will also be sharing supporting resources for the book on our website, www.upfitness.com

 @UPFITNESS   @UPFITNESSLIVE   /LONDONPERSONALTRAINERS

SETTING UP FOR SUCCESS

SETTING UP FOR SUCCESS
ESTABLISH YOUR STARTING POINT

The first step in setting up for success is to establish your starting point.

To do this, you will complete the same body composition assessment that we use with clients in their first session at Ultimate Performance.

The assessment involves:

▶ Recording your bodyweight.

▶ Taking circumference measurements.

▶ Taking progress pictures
(the infamous 'before' and 'after' pictures).

▶ Estimating your body fat percentage.

The body composition assessment is a vital part of your transformation.

Seeing your starting pictures and measurements can inspire you to take action, and once you are up and running, watching your body take shape and the numbers drop can be equally rewarding.

It also serves a very practical purpose, as you will use the results to create your meal plan and inform any changes you need to make based on your progress.

We have provided comprehensive guides on how to complete each stage of the assessment in the *'Progress Assessment'* section.

Each guide covers:

▶ Equipment requirements.

▶ Recommended frequency and timing of measurement.

▶ How to perform the assessment.

▶ Key issues and trainer tips.

You can read ahead but make sure to schedule time to complete the baseline assessment, as you will need the results to create your meal plan.

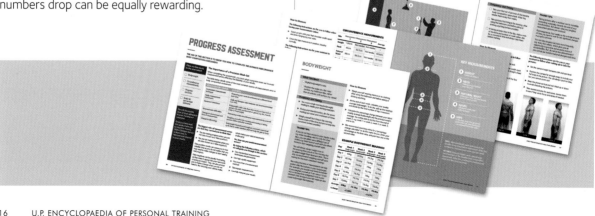

TRANSFORMATION TIME FRAMES

WHY WE RECOMMEND 12 WEEKS

We recommend putting aside 12 weeks to complete your transformation.

From experience, this is the longest time people can commit to before needing a break. An unavoidable truth about transformation programs is that they require a level of discipline and attention to detail that many of your friends, family and colleagues may struggle to understand.

You can sustain a highly focused approach for a relatively short period, but not indefinitely. Nobody is a robot.

YOU MAY NEED LESS THAN 12 WEEKS

If you are starting from a relatively lean position, you may be able to achieve your body composition goals in less than 12 weeks.

However, unless you are an experienced dieter, you have no way of knowing for sure how long you will need. It takes several cycles of dieting to get a solid understanding of how long you need to reach a given body fat percentage. Life can get in the way and affect your ability to follow the plan, for example, travel, social commitments or even the flu!

It is better to overestimate how long you need and then end your diet in advance of the 12 weeks if you achieve your target look ahead of time.

YOU MAY NEED MORE THAN 12 WEEKS

There is a limit to how much body fat you can lose in 12 weeks and some people may need more time to achieve their long-term body composition goals.

If this is the case, we recommend taking a break from dieting after week 12 to focus on consolidating your results. Following this, you can then undertake another block of transformation dieting.

How long you should break for between each dieting phase depends on the length of the initial diet, how much longer you want to diet for and practical issues like aligning the next diet with your schedule.

When attempting large scale body composition changes, breaking it up into more manageable chunks makes it less daunting and from experience leads to more sustainable results.

YOU MAY HAVE LESS THAN 12 WEEKS

If your goal date is less than 12 weeks away, it is still possible to get in great shape, but you will have to tailor your expectations about what is realistically achievable.

There is always the option to make your impending goal date a short-term target and continue to diet afterwards in pursuit of a more long-term goal.

SCHEDULING YOUR TRANSFORMATION

TRANSFORMATION START AND END DATES

When scheduling your transformation, we strongly recommend aligning your start and end dates with a specific occasion where you want to look your best.

Without a clear start and end date, most dieters struggle to stay motivated and ultimately never achieve their goals.

A prime example of this are the countless people who embark upon post-Christmas diets with the vague goal to 'lose some weight'. In most cases, the diet is no longer in place come February. Now, compare this to a future bride preparing for her wedding day or somebody wanting to make a big impression at their college reunion - nothing will get in their way!

Some obvious dates to target include holidays and special events like birthdays and weddings.

If you do not have a specific goal but just the clear idea of wanting a transformation, you should seriously consider creating one. For example, several of our clients have found it extremely motivating to book a photoshoot or holiday to mark the end of their transformation.

Having a motivational goal date gives you something tangible to aim for and keeps you accountable when times get tough.

WITHOUT A CLEAR START AND END DATE, MOST DIETERS STRUGGLE TO STAY MOTIVATED AND ULTIMATELY NEVER ACHIEVE THEIR GOALS.

SELECTING YOUR START AND END DATES

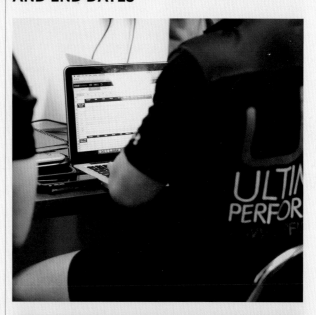

 ACTION:
Before continuing, choose your start and motivational end dates and mark them on your calendar.

We have highlighted some example periods that are conducive to dieting and some that are less so on the diagram opposite.

For now, only focus on scheduling your first 12 weeks (or less, if targeting a more short-term date), even if you think you may need longer.

During your diet break, you can review your progress and decide if this is a temporary break or a more permanent return to maintenance.

JANUARY

S	M	T	W	T	F	S
	1	2	3	4	5	6
7	8	9	10	11	12	13
14	15	16	17	18	19	20
21	22	23	24	25	26	27
28	29	30	31			

FEBRUARY

S	M	T	W	T	F	S
				1	2	3
4	5	6	7	8	9	10
11	12	13	14	15	16	17
18	19	20	21	22	23	24
25	26	27	28			

MARCH

S	M	T	W	T	F	S
				1	2	3
4	5	6	7	8	9	10
11	12	13	14	15	16	17
18	19	20	21	22	23	24
25	26	27	28	29	30	31

APRIL

S	M	T	W	T	F	S
1	2	3	4	5	6	7
8	9	10	11	12	13	14
15	16	17	18	19	20	21
22	23	24	25	26	27	28
29	30					

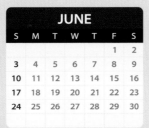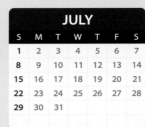

WINTER | **SPRING**

JANUARY / NEW YEAR
Most people will be dieting so there will be fewer temptations and more social support.

SPRING
Start here and be lean for summer!

MAY

S	M	T	W	T	F	S
		1	2	3	4	5
6	7	8	9	10	11	12
13	14	15	16	17	18	19
20	21	22	23	24	25	26
27	28	29	30	31		

JUNE

S	M	T	W	T	F	S
					1	2
3	4	5	6	7	8	9
10	11	12	13	14	15	16
17	18	19	20	21	22	23
24	25	26	27	28	29	30

JULY

S	M	T	W	T	F	S
1	2	3	4	5	6	7
8	9	10	11	12	13	14
15	16	17	18	19	20	21
22	23	24	25	26	27	28
29	30	31				

AUGUST

S	M	T	W	T	F	S
			1	2	3	4
5	6	7	8	9	10	11
12	13	14	15	16	17	18
19	20	21	22	23	24	25
26	27	28	29	30	31	

SUMMER

RELIGIOUS EVENTS
e.g. Ramadan.

SUMMER
Be aware of holidays and social events like parties and weddings.

SEPTEMBER

S	M	T	W	T	F	S
						1
2	3	4	5	6	7	8
9	10	11	12	13	14	15
16	17	18	19	20	21	22
23	24	25	26	27	28	29
30						

OCTOBER

S	M	T	W	T	F	S
	1	2	3	4	5	6
7	8	9	10	11	12	13
14	15	16	17	18	19	20
21	22	23	24	25	26	27
28	29	30	31			

NOVEMBER

S	M	T	W	T	F	S
				1	2	3
4	5	6	7	8	9	10
11	12	13	14	15	16	17
18	19	20	21	22	23	24
25	26	27	28	29	30	

DECEMBER

S	M	T	W	T	F	S
						1
2	3	4	5	6	7	8
9	10	11	12	13	14	15
16	17	18	19	20	21	22
23	24	25	26	27	28	29
30	31					

AUTUMN

AUTUMN
Normally quiet, but the Christmas party season starts earlier each year.

WINTER
Lots of social events to navigate like work Christmas parties.

MOTIVATIONAL GOAL DATES
Example motivational dates to target: Milestone birthdays, e.g. 30th or 40th / Weddings / Holidays / Photoshoots.

THE 12 WEEK REVIEW

Once you have identified your start and end dates, the next step is to review your transformation time frame and identify any events that will affect your ability to follow your training and meal plan.

Common examples include:

▶ **Travel**, e.g. business and pleasure.

▶ **Stressful periods**, e.g. work, family and exams.

▶ **Special occasions**, e.g. birthdays and anniversaries.

▶ **Social events**, e.g. nights out with friends.

No 12 week period will ever be without some challenges and now is the best time to work out how to overcome these potentially derailing events. Performing this review will address any major events and you can deal with less significant ones that crop up as part of your weekly meal planning.

We have outlined several methods you can use to adjust your approach to stay on track in the 'Transformation Meal Planning' section.

SCHEDULE PROGRESS CHECK-INS

You will repeat each part of the body composition assessment protocol several times throughout your transformation.

Specifically, you need to schedule time and set reminders to:

▶ Measure your bodyweight each morning.

▶ Take your circumference measurements each week.

▶ Review your progress at the end of each week to see if you are on target or need to make changes.

▶ Take progress pictures every 2-4 weeks. For more details, see the 'Progress Assessment' section.

EXTRA CONSIDERATIONS – THE PRACTICE WEEK

Jumping straight into a transformation program can be overwhelming, especially if you are new to the approaches outlined in this book.

One strategy you can use to make the transition less abrupt is to schedule a practice week before starting your full-blown transformation program.

Even experienced dieters can benefit from an adjustment period if they have spent the last few months being more flexible with their approach to nutrition.

ONE STRATEGY YOU CAN USE TO MAKE THE TRANSITION LESS ABRUPT IS TO SCHEDULE A PRACTICE WEEK BEFORE STARTING YOUR FULL-BLOWN TRANSFORMATION PROGRAM.

Here is a list of example activities you can perform in the practice week

☐ Complete the baseline body composition assessment (p.88).

☐ Find a diet partner (p.21).

☐ Design or select a resistance training program to follow (p.22).

☐ Download and practice using a nutrition tracking application (p.62).

☐ Start recording your daily step total and morning bodyweight (p.89).

12-WEEK REVIEW

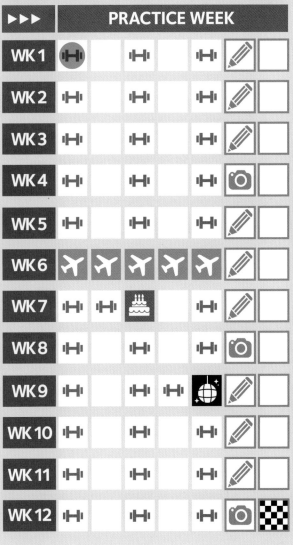

PRACTICE WEEK

▶▶▶							
WK 1	●		🏋		🏋	✏	
WK 2	🏋		🏋		🏋	✏	
WK 3	🏋		🏋		🏋	✏	
WK 4	🏋		🏋		🏋	📷	
WK 5	🏋		🏋		🏋	✏	
WK 6	✈	✈	✈	✈	✈	✏	
WK 7	🏋	🏋	🎂		🏋	✏	
WK 8	🏋		🏋		🏋	📷	
WK 9	🏋		🏋	🏋	🪩	✏	
WK 10	🏋		🏋		🏋	✏	
WK 11	🏋		🏋		🏋	✏	
WK 12	🏋		🏋		🏋	📷	🏁

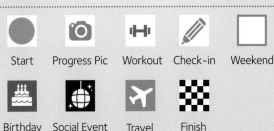

● Start	📷 Progress Pic	🏋 Workout	✏ Check-in	☐ Weekend
🎂 Birthday	🪩 Social Event (e.g. night out)	✈ Travel (Holiday)	🏁 Finish	

EXTRA CONSIDERATIONS – DIET PARTNER

A key part of a client's transformation journey at Ultimate Performance is the daily contact (in person and online) with their trainer and the accountability this provides.

You can recreate this for yourself by asking a friend or family member to be your diet partner. This can be somebody who wants to diet at the same time or who is just willing to keep you accountable.

You can even raise the stakes by making a 'diet bet' with your diet partner, for example, agreeing a forfeit for every missed check-in.

> ⚠ **ACTION:**
> At the end of each day, message your diet partner with the following information:

● ● ●   **Compose message**

To: john.doe@support.com

Subject: Andrew's daily check-in 1st January

- Morning bodyweight, *e.g. 80kg.*

- Daily step total, *e.g. 10,000 steps.*

- Training summary, *e.g. upper body workout.*

- Food diary, *e.g. screenshot from a food tracking application or written record.*

Attachments: *MyFitnessPal Food Diary Screenshot'*

Send

TRANSFORMATION TRAINING

ALTHOUGH THE FOCUS OF THIS BOOK IS ON NUTRITION, WE CANNOT IGNORE THE IMPORTANT CONTRIBUTION THAT TRAINING AND REGULAR PHYSICAL ACTIVITY MAKE IN TRANSFORMING YOUR BODY COMPOSITION.

This section will explain the role of each type of activity in your transformation program and outline our recommendations.

RESISTANCE TRAINING

Resistance training is a type of exercise that forces your muscles to work against resistance provided by your own bodyweight, free weights (dumbbells and barbells) and machines.

When restricting calories to lose body fat, there is a risk that you will lose muscle. This is known as low-quality weight loss and reinforces why losing scale weight should not be your primary goal on a transformation program.

Research has consistently shown that resistance training in combination with a high-protein diet can maintain or even increase muscle mass during periods of caloric restriction.

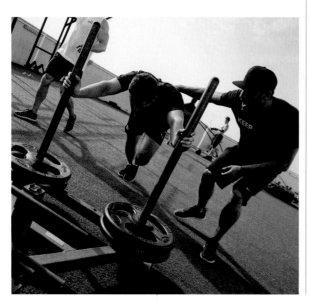

Resistance Training Recommendations

For the best results, we recommend resistance training three to four times a week.

Training Frequency: 3 x Per Week

If you choose to train three times per week, we recommend alternating between two full-body workouts.

Using a full body program will allow you to train each muscle group at least twice per week, which research suggests is the optimal training frequency for muscle growth.

After you have completed each workout 6-8 times, you will need to update both workouts by making changes to program design variables, such as exercise selection and the number of sets and reps.

	3 Workouts Week 1	3 Workouts Week 2
Mon	Full Body Workout A	Full Body Workout B
Tue	–	–
Wed	Full Body Workout B	Full Body Workout A
Thu	–	–
Fri	Full Body Workout A	Full Body Workout B
Sat	–	–
Sun	–	–

Training Frequency: 4 x Per Week

If you choose to train four times per week, you can either use a full body approach or split your program into upper body and lower body workouts.

Repeat each workout twice per week until you have completed each one 6-8 times and then update both workouts.

Only choose the upper/lower body training split option if you are confident that you can consistently train four times per week.

TRY TO AVOID TRAINING ON THREE CONSECUTIVE DAYS TO GIVE YOUR BODY TIME TO RECOVER, ALTHOUGH THIS IS BETTER THAN NOT TRAINING AT ALL AND WILL NOT AFFECT YOUR RESULTS IF YOU ARE GENERALLY ON TOP OF RECOVERY.

	OPTION 1 4 Workouts (Upper/Lower)	OPTION 2 4 Workouts (Full Body)
Mon	Upper Body Workout	Full Body Workout A
Tue	Lower Body Workout	Full Body Workout B
Wed	–	–
Thu	Upper Body Workout	Full Body Workout A
Fri	Lower Body Workout	Full Body Workout B
Sat	–	–
Sun	–	–

Try to avoid training on three consecutive days to give your body time to recover, although this is better than not training at all and will not affect your results if you are generally on top of recovery (nutrition, sleep and stress management).

We have provided sample workouts and review program design in more detail in the companion book, *'Principles of Muscle Building Program Design'*.

NON-EXERCISE ACTIVITY THERMOGENESIS (NEAT)

From a calorie-burning perspective, how physically active you are outside of the gym can have a real impact on your fat loss efforts.

The technical term for how many calories you burn outside of the gym is non-exercise activity thermogenesis (NEAT for short).

Part of NEAT is voluntary and largely determined by your occupation and how you choose to spend your leisure time. There is also an involuntary component beyond your conscious control that you generate from maintaining your posture and small bodily movements known as fidgeting.

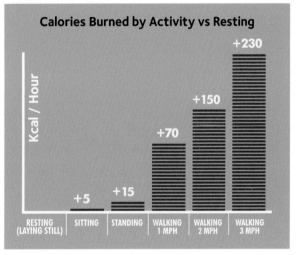

Adapted from Levine (2007).

The Importance of An Active Lifestyle

The diagram above shows the calories burned performing several activities.

Sit down for an hour, and you will burn roughly 5kcal more than you would laying down still. Stand up and this triples to 15kcal more per hour. Start walking and you can burn up to 230kcal more per hour.

While the exact values will vary depending on your bodyweight and how vigorously you move, these figures highlight how simply moving around more has the potential to add up to a surprisingly large calorie count over the course of a day.

In fact, Dr James Levine of the Mayo Clinic estimates that we have lost up to 2,000kcal of activity from our day in the transition to becoming a mainly sedentary society – a full day's worth of eating for a lot of people!

How Active Are You?

A simple test to evaluate your NEAT levels is to use your mobile phone or pedometer to track how many steps you take during a typical day.

The table below shows the number of steps we consider to be representative of a sedentary and active lifestyle.

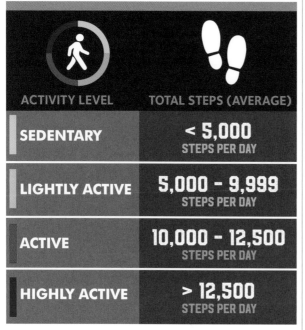

ACTIVITY LEVEL	TOTAL STEPS (AVERAGE)
SEDENTARY	< 5,000 STEPS PER DAY
LIGHTLY ACTIVE	5,000 – 9,999 STEPS PER DAY
ACTIVE	10,000 – 12,500 STEPS PER DAY
HIGHLY ACTIVE	> 12,500 STEPS PER DAY

If you currently take less than 10,000 steps, you will benefit from making changes to your routine to become more active.

On top of several health benefits, you will be less dependent on caloric restriction to lose body fat and will be able to diet on a higher number of calories.

Numerous research studies have also shown NEAT (mainly the involuntary component) to decline in response to weight loss as an attempt by the body to conserve energy during periods of low energy availability.

ON TOP OF SEVERAL HEALTH BENEFITS, YOU WILL BE LESS DEPENDENT ON CALORIC RESTRICTION TO LOSE BODY FAT AND WILL BE ABLE TO DIET ON A HIGHER NUMBER OF CALORIES.

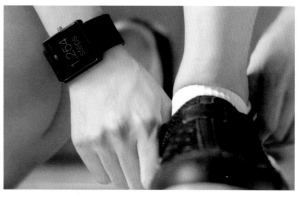

This is a natural part of weight loss and simply your body doing its job, ensuring you have enough energy to keep going. Making an effort to keep voluntary components of NEAT high can help offset this adaptive reduction and prevent fat loss plateaus.

NEAT Recommendations

Walking is the main component of most people's NEAT, and you can track your step count using your mobile phone or pedometer.

Aim for a minimum average step target of 10,000 steps.

The target is an average so you can make up for low-step days, such as long-distance travel, with more active days later in the week.

Where possible, aim for 'active steps', for example, making it a rule to take the stairs or walking at a brisk pace.

If you already take more than 10,000 steps as part of your normal routine, aim to keep this consistent.

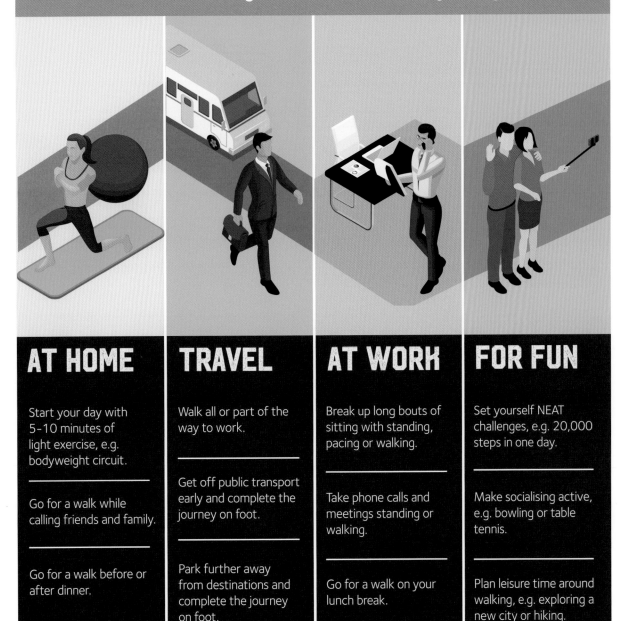

If you currently take less than 10,000 steps, try some of the following ideas to build NEAT into your day:

AT HOME

Start your day with 5-10 minutes of light exercise, e.g. bodyweight circuit.

Go for a walk while calling friends and family.

Go for a walk before or after dinner.

TRAVEL

Walk all or part of the way to work.

Get off public transport early and complete the journey on foot.

Park further away from destinations and complete the journey on foot.

AT WORK

Break up long bouts of sitting with standing, pacing or walking.

Take phone calls and meetings standing or walking.

Go for a walk on your lunch break.

FOR FUN

Set yourself NEAT challenges, e.g. 20,000 steps in one day.

Make socialising active, e.g. bowling or table tennis.

Plan leisure time around walking, e.g. exploring a new city or hiking.

By the way, do not pay much attention to the calorie burn estimates provided by commercial grade activity trackers. While they are great awareness tools, the algorithms are not accurate enough to manage your calorie intake.

FORMAL CARDIO

Formal cardio refers to structured workouts performed as part of your training program with a specific goal, for example:

▶ Develop cardiovascular fitness.

▶ Offset an otherwise sedentary lifestyle.

▶ Burn calories.

There are three main types of formal cardio that are identifiable based on training intensity (how hard you work) which you can measure using the following rate of perceived exertion (RPE) scale.

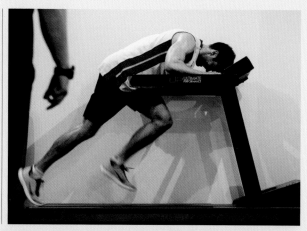

RATE OF PERCEIVED EXERTION (RPE) SCALE		
RPE SCALE	**EMOJI**	**WHAT THIS FEELS LIKE...**
9-10	😵	**MAX EFFORT** – This pace should feel as if it is almost impossible to keep going. You will be out of breath and unable to talk.
7-8	😓	**CHALLENGING** – This pace should feel difficult to maintain and you will only be able to speak a few words.
5-6	🙁	**MODERATELY CHALLENGING** – This pace should feel uncomfortable and you will only be able to hold a short conversation.
3-4	😀	**EASY** – This pace should feel as if you can keep going for hours, while holding a full conversation.
1-2	🙂	**VERY EASY** – This pace should feel like very little effort, but more than not moving at all.

LOW-INTENSITY STEADY STATE (LISS)

Low-intensity activity (RPE 1-4) maintained for extended periods of time, e.g. incline treadmill walking for 30-minutes.

MODERATE-INTENSITY STEADY STATE (MISS)

Moderate-intensity activity (RPE 5-6) maintained for extended periods of time, e.g. 5km run.

HIGH-INTENSITY INTERVAL TRAINING (HIIT)

Alternates short periods of high-intensity exercise (RPE 7-10) with less-intense recovery periods (RPE 1-4), e.g. alternating between sprinting and walking.

We also consider most group fitness classes, e.g. spinning and circuit training, to be versions of HIIT training.

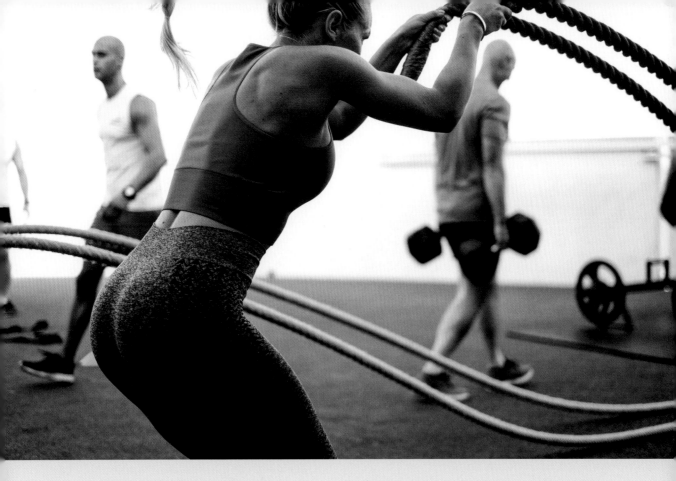

Always Prioritise Resistance Training

If you can only get to the gym three times a week and have no other opportunities to train, then resistance training should always take priority over formal cardio.

You can develop your fitness, lose body fat and avoid a sedentary lifestyle by sticking to your diet and keeping active outside of the gym. In contrast, lifting weights is the only way to build muscle.

IF YOU CAN ONLY GET TO THE GYM THREE TIMES A WEEK AND HAVE NO OTHER OPPORTUNITIES TO TRAIN, THEN RESISTANCE TRAINING SHOULD ALWAYS TAKE PRIORITY OVER FORMAL CARDIO.

However, there are several physical and practical benefits associated with formal cardio:

1. MISS and HIIT both develop your work capacity which can have a beneficial impact on your resistance training.

2. Formal cardio develops mental toughness.

3. If short on time and low on steps, performing a MISS or HIIT workout can boost your daily physical activity levels in a time-efficient manner.

4. Many of our clients enjoy performing formal cardio, particularly the group element of fitness classes.

5. The low skill component lets beginner trainees push themselves harder than they can while lifting weights.

LISS vs MISS vs HIIT

The intensity level of the different formal cardio options can have a significant impact on their compatibility with resistance training.

LISS is not intense enough to interfere with your recovery from or performance in resistance training workouts. The primary role of LISS in a training program is to burn additional calories. You can use LISS to help meet your daily step target, for example, walking on the treadmill for 10 minutes before your resistance training workout – this is also a great mental warm-up!

The main issue to be aware of with MISS is that your body adapts specifically to the types of training that you perform. The problem this poses is that resistance training and MISS place opposite and competing demands on your body.

Resistance training conditions your muscles to lift heavy weights explosively and for short durations, whereas MISS conditions your muscles to work at lower intensities for longer durations.

This should not be a problem if you limit the amount of MISS performed. However, you can avoid the issue altogether by using HIIT instead.

The high-intensity nature of HIIT and time spent working versus resting is very similar to resistance training, which results in complementary rather than competing adaptations.

For example, sprinting flat out for 30 seconds and then resting for 90 seconds is comparable to lifting a heavy weight for 10 reps and then resting for an equivalent amount of time.

RESISTANCE TRAINING CONDITIONS YOUR MUSCLES TO LIFT HEAVY WEIGHTS EXPLOSIVELY AND FOR SHORT DURATIONS, WHEREAS MISS CONDITIONS YOUR MUSCLES TO WORK AT LOWER INTENSITIES FOR LONGER DURATIONS.

You Have a Limited Recovery Capacity

There is a limit to how much training you can recover from, and both MISS and HIIT add to the total amount of exercise-related stress placed on your body. Remember, any cardio you do takes place in the same week that you will also be resistance training three to four times.

Formal Cardio Recommendations

If you are training three to four times a week and meeting your NEAT target, you do not need to include a formal cardio component in your training program.

Perform a maximum of two cardio workouts (MISS or HIIT) per week if resistance training three times.

Perform a maximum of one cardio workout (MISS or HIIT) per week if resistance training four times.

There is no limit for LISS cardio as this does not challenge your body enough to interfere with recovery or workout performance.

Always perform cardio after resistance training if doing both on the same day. However, the ideal time to complete cardio workouts is on a non-resistance training day.

You can find sample formal cardio workouts in the companion book, *'Principles of Muscle Building Program Design'*.

	3 Workouts Per Week	4 Workouts Per Week
Mon	Workout 1	Workout 1
Tue	Cardio Workout	Workout 2
Wed	Workout 2	*Rest Day*
Thu	*Rest Day*	Workout 3
Fri	Workout 3	Workout 4
Sat	Cardio Workout	Cardio Workout
Sun	*Rest Day*	*Rest Day*

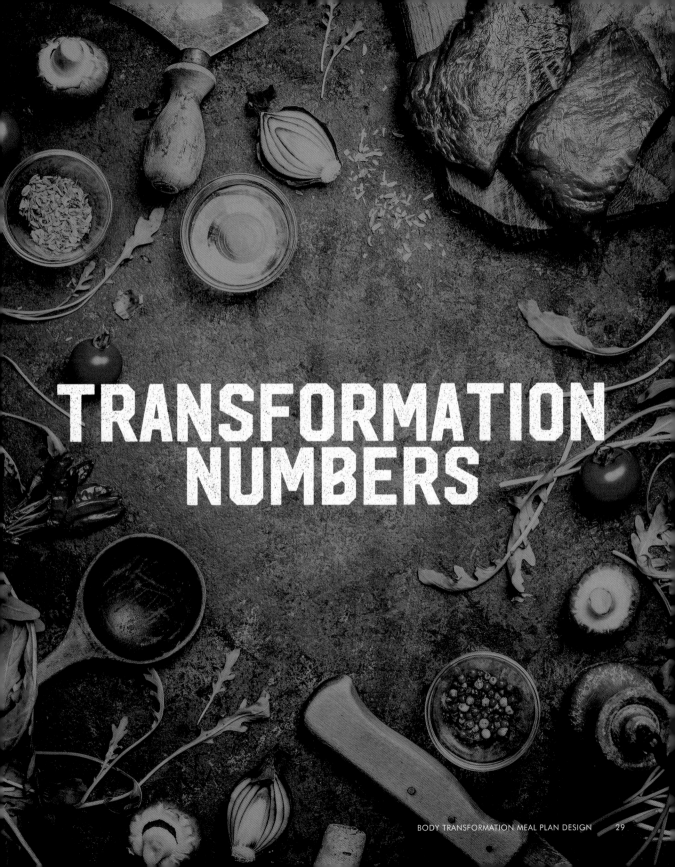

TRANSFORMATION NUMBERS

TRANSFORMATION NUMBERS
HOW TO CALCULATE YOUR NUTRITION TARGETS

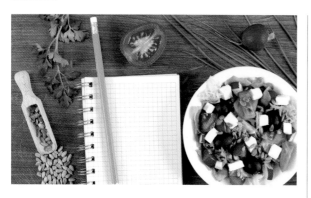

NOW THAT YOU HAVE SET UP FOR SUCCESS, THE NEXT STEP IS TO CALCULATE THE NUTRITION TARGETS THAT YOU WILL USE TO CREATE YOUR MEAL PLAN.

To do this, you will follow a three-step process which we have outlined in the diagram opposite.

Make sure you have completed the body composition assessment, as you will need the following information to complete the calculations:

▶ 1 x morning bodyweight reading.
▶ Body fat percentage estimate.

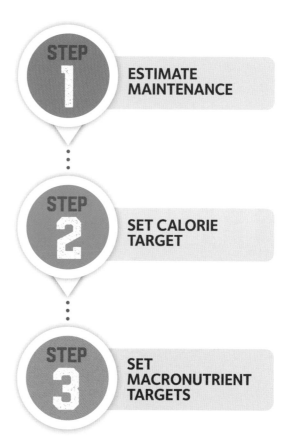

STEP 1 — ESTIMATE MAINTENANCE

STEP 2 — SET CALORIE TARGET

STEP 3 — SET MACRONUTRIENT TARGETS

WANT TO SKIP THE MATHS?

If you want to skip the maths, we have provided pre-calculated nutrition targets in the *'Quick Start Nutrition Targets'* section (p.187).

Simply, find the appropriate nutrition targets for your bodyweight and body fat percentage in the reference tables, and progress to *'Transformation Foods'* to start creating your meal plan.

STEP 1: ESTIMATE MAINTENANCE

WHAT IS MAINTENANCE AND WHY START HERE?

The starting point for setting your calorie target is to figure out how many calories you need to consume to maintain your current bodyweight.

The number of calories this equates to is known as your maintenance calorie intake, or more technically, your total daily energy expenditure (TDEE).

TDEE consists of three components:

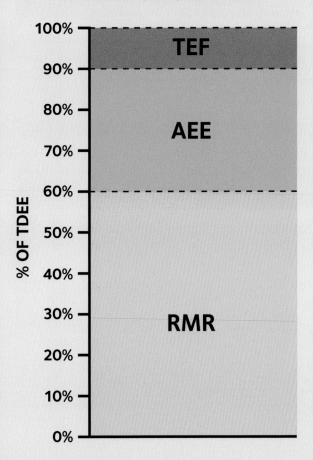

TOTAL DAILY ENERGY EXPENDITURE (TDEE) BREAKDOWN

Resting Metabolic Rate (RMR)

▶ RMR is the minimum amount of energy your body needs to maintain vital life functions at rest, such as your heart rate and breathing.

▶ RMR accounts for 50-70% of the average person's TDEE.

▶ Why 50-70%? Because the exact value depends on how physically active you are. If you suddenly become more active and increase your TDEE, then your RMR will account for a smaller percentage.

Thermic Effect of Food (TEF)

▶ TEF is the number of calories you burn digesting, absorbing and processing foods for use and storage inside your body.

▶ Each macronutrient (protein, fat and carbohydrate) has a different thermic effect:

Protein	Fat	Carbohydrate
20-30%	1-3%	5-10%

▶ As you can see, it costs your body a lot more energy to digest and absorb protein-rich foods. For every 100kcal of protein you consume, your body burns 20-30kcal processing them.

▶ A commonly used estimate is that TEF accounts for 10% of your total calorie intake assuming a balanced diet. For example, if you eat 2,000kcal per day, then you will burn 200kcal processing your meals.

▶ This does not mean that spreading your daily calorie intake over a greater number of meals will burn more calories or 'stoke your metabolism'. TEF will be the same regardless of whether you eat three or six meals if the total calories consumed are the same. Eating more frequently will just result in more regular, but smaller, thermic effects compared to eating fewer larger meals.

Activity Energy Expenditure (AEE)

▶ AEE is the number of calories you burn performing purposeful exercise (resistance training and formal cardio) and all other physical activity that is not sleeping or eating.

▶ AEE ranges from 15% of TDEE in sedentary individuals up to 50% in highly active individuals.

The reason we start by estimating your maintenance calorie intake is that you need to set your calorie target below this to lose body fat.

When this happens, you create a calorie deficit which forces your body to mobilise stored energy in the form of body fat and lean body mass (LBM) to help meet your daily energy requirements.

Obviously, the goal is to use body fat, not LBM, to overcome the calorie deficit which you can signal your body to do by resistance training and eating a high-protein diet.

Without an accurate estimate of maintenance, you risk setting your calorie target too high and creating a calorie surplus where it is impossible to lose body fat.

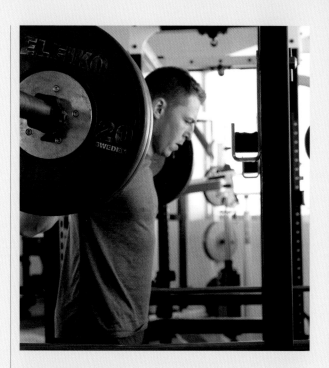

THE REASON WE START BY ESTIMATING YOUR MAINTENANCE CALORIE INTAKE IS THAT YOU NEED TO SET YOUR CALORIE TARGET BELOW THIS TO LOSE BODY FAT.

Calorie Intake	Calorie Balance	Status	Effect
Below maintenance (calorie deficit)	Negative calorie balance	Breakdown mode	Stored calories (body fat and LBM) burned
Maintenance	Neutral	Maintenance mode	No change in energy stores
Above maintenance (calorie surplus)	Positive calorie balance	Storage mode	Surplus calories stored as body fat and LBM

Note: Your body's primary LBM energy stores are muscle mass, other body proteins and glycogen (the storage form of carbohydrate in the body).

How to Estimate Your Maintenance

A key point to understand about your maintenance calorie intake is that it is not a fixed value. Instead, it is more appropriate to think of it as a moving target that can change from one day to the next.

Although your RMR stays relatively stable over time, your activity levels can vary significantly from one day to the next.

As an extreme example, an athlete who trains for several hours a day may need to eat 4,000kcal (think, three large pizzas) to maintain their current bodyweight.

Imagine if they broke a leg in training. If this happened, their maintenance calorie intake would cut in half overnight as they would be lying in a hospital bed unable to move. If they continued to eat 4,000kcal, they would gain a lot of body fat!

Less extreme examples include being more active on weekends compared to weekdays or walking instead of driving to work on some days.

Whatever the cause, the reality is that you will almost never burn the same number of calories each day. The difference between days can be a little or a lot depending on how consistent your activity levels are.

A KEY POINT TO UNDERSTAND ABOUT YOUR MAINTENANCE CALORIE INTAKE IS THAT IT IS NOT A FIXED VALUE. INSTEAD, IT IS MORE APPROPRIATE TO THINK OF IT AS A MOVING TARGET THAT CAN CHANGE FROM ONE DAY TO THE NEXT.

The Tracking Method

The most reliable and surprisingly low-tech way to determine your maintenance calorie intake is to record your calorie intake in a food diary and monitor changes in your bodyweight over time.

You can then estimate your maintenance calorie intake based on how much weight you gain or lose (if any) during the tracking period:

▶ If your bodyweight increases, then on average your calorie intake was above your maintenance calorie level.

▶ If your bodyweight decreases, then on average your calorie intake was below your maintenance calorie level.

▶ If your bodyweight stays roughly the same, then on average your calorie intake was equal to your maintenance calorie level.

The advantage of the tracking method is that it smooths out any daily fluctuations and allows you to estimate your maintenance calorie intake based on trends in your activity levels over time.

The Problems with The Tracking Method...

We tend not to use the tracking method at the start of a transformation diet because:

▶ It delays the start of your transformation by at least two weeks. Any less than this and daily fluctuations in bodyweight (caused by food weight and water retention) can skew your results.

▶ Most people tend to clean up their diet and eat fewer calories when they start tracking their calorie intake, which can also trigger bodyweight fluctuations.

▶ Nutrition tracking is a skill. If you are new to tracking or out of practice, then you are more likely to misreport your calorie intake at the start of a diet.

From experience, the best time to use the tracking method is at the end of your transformation, when you have more experience of tracking your nutrition, a rough idea of what your maintenance calorie intake may be and more time for trial and error.

Note: we discuss bodyweight fluctuations in more detail in the 'Progress Assessment' section.

The Solution: The Calculation Method

The alternative to the tracking method, and our preferred starting point, is the calculation method.

This approach involves using a simple two-step calculation to estimate your maintenance calorie intake, which we will guide you through in the following section.

Before continuing, we need to stress that the calculations are based on scientific research findings and textbook theory that are not specific to you as an individual.

As a result, the nutrition targets you start your transformation with are not magic and guaranteed to work.

Instead, they will always be somewhat of an educated 'best guess' that you may need to adjust based on your progress.

This highlights the importance of accurate progress assessment and knowing when and how to make changes, which we explain in detail in the *'How to Make Changes'* section.

CALCULATION #1:
Estimate Resting Metabolic Rate (RMR)

You can test your RMR with an extremely high degree of accuracy by visiting the sports science department at your local university, but this is expensive and impractical for the purposes of creating a meal plan.

Instead, you can use one of several prediction equations that researchers have developed based on the relationship between RMR and more easily measured variables like your LBM, height, age and gender.

We recommend using the 'Katch-McArdle formula' which is based on your LBM and weight in kilograms.

Various online calculators will complete the formula for you, but you can also work it out for yourself using the following guide.

We have provided examples of how to complete all the transformation number calculations at the end of this section.

HOW TO CALCULATE YOUR RESTING METABOLIC RATE

STEP 1:
CONVERT BODYWEIGHT INTO KILOGRAMS

The Katch-McArdle formula uses kilograms, so if you usually measure in pounds, you need to make the conversion. To do this, divide your bodyweight in pounds by 2.2 (2.2lb = 1kg).

STEP 2:
CALCULATE HOW MUCH BODY FAT YOU HAVE

Now use the body fat percentage estimate you calculated as part of your baseline body composition assessment to work out how much body fat you have in kilograms (fat mass).

STARTING BODYWEIGHT (KG)	X	BODY FAT PERCENTAGE % (in decimal form)

To convert your body fat percentage into decimal form, you need to divide it by 100.

20% becomes 0.2, 25% becomes 0.25, and so on.

STEP 3:
CALCULATE YOUR LBM

STARTING BODYWEIGHT (KG)	–	FAT MASS (KG)

STEP 4:
COMPLETE THE KATCH-MCARDLE FORMULA

KATCH-MCARDLE FORMULA	=	(21.6 X LBM KG) + 370

You need to break the formula into two parts:
Part 1: 21.6 x LBM KG
Part 2: 'Part 1 answer' + 370

CALCULATION #2:
Apply Activity Multiplier

Once you have estimated your RMR, the next step is to factor in your activity energy expenditure (AEE).

The concept behind activity multipliers is simple. Select an appropriate multiplier for your activity levels and apply it to your RMR to estimate your maintenance calorie intake.

How to Estimate Your Activity Levels

An activity multiplier of 'x 1' is impossible as all bodily movement requires energy. So, your maintenance calorie intake will always be higher than your RMR. As soon as you get out of bed, you are burning calories above a resting level.

For context, researchers have recorded physical activity levels as high as 4.5 times RMR in competitive cyclists and arctic explorers, and as low as 1.2 in hospital patients.

As a result, some major twists of fate could potentially see somebody with an RMR of 2,000kcal burn as little as 2,400kcal or up to 9,000kcal per day.

However, these extremes in activity are not sustainable in the long-term, and from experience, most people will fall somewhere between 1.4 and 2.2.

A common mistake people make at this stage of the set-up process is obsessing over which activity multiplier best represents their lifestyle.

This is partly due to most exercise textbooks being frustratingly vague in their descriptions, for example, defining an active lifestyle as 'moderate exercise 3-5 times per week'.

The truth is that estimating your activity levels is not an exact science.

The aim is to find a reasonable starting point that does not grossly-under or overestimate your maintenance calorie intake. You can then make adjustments based on how your body responds in the early stages of your diet.

As a result, we recommend selecting an activity multiplier of 'x 1.5'.

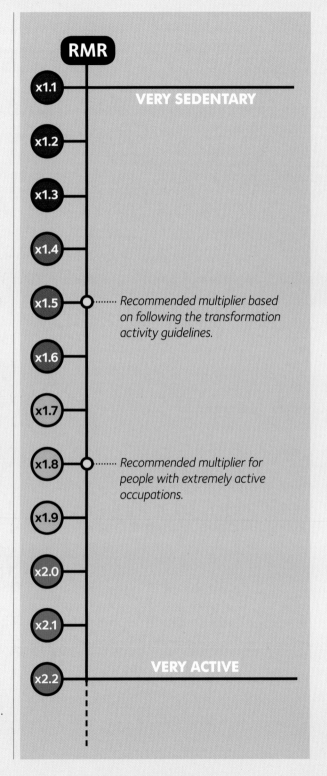

RMR

x1.1
x1.2
x1.3
x1.4
x1.5 .... *Recommended multiplier based on following the transformation activity guidelines.*
x1.6
x1.7
x1.8 .... *Recommended multiplier for people with extremely active occupations.*
x1.9
x2.0
x2.1
x2.2

VERY SEDENTARY

VERY ACTIVE

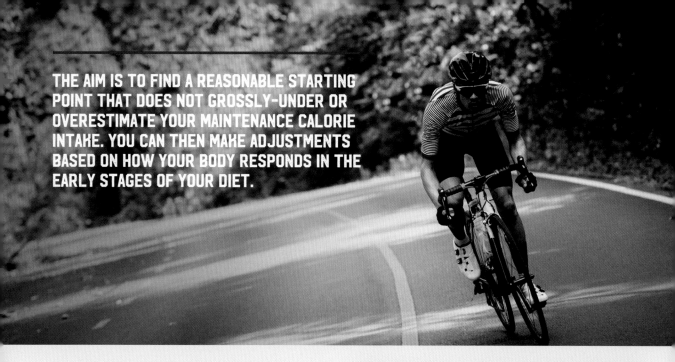

THE AIM IS TO FIND A REASONABLE STARTING POINT THAT DOES NOT GROSSLY-UNDER OR OVERESTIMATE YOUR MAINTENANCE CALORIE INTAKE. YOU CAN THEN MAKE ADJUSTMENTS BASED ON HOW YOUR BODY RESPONDS IN THE EARLY STAGES OF YOUR DIET.

It is important to note that this is based on the assumption that you will be following the transformation activity guidelines outlined in the *'Setting Up for Success'* section.

The one exception to this is if you have an extremely active occupation that involves day-long physically active work. For example, a construction worker or farmer.

If this is the case, we recommend selecting an activity multiplier of 'x 1.8'.

Extremely active occupations are becoming increasingly rare, but it is a lot more common for people to have jobs with variable activity levels. For example, personal trainers, estate agents and shop assistants can all have busy and quiet days.

If this is the case, only select 'x 1.8' if you anticipate consistently having more busy than quiet days during your transformation, i.e. four or more extremely active days each week.

If you are unsure about which option to select, go with 'x 1.5' and you can always make adjustments based on your progress.

HOW TO APPLY YOUR ACTIVITY MULTIPLIER

Select your activity multiplier and use the following formula to estimate your maintenance calorie intake:

RMR	X	ACTIVITY MULTIPLIER

What About Thermic Effect of Food (TEF)?

The final factor to consider is the thermic effect of food, which if you recall is the amount of energy you expend digesting and processing food for use and storage.

While you can multiply your current maintenance value by 1.1 to get a crude estimate (TEF = 10% of calorie intake), because TEF makes up a relatively small part of your TDEE we typically exclude it from our calculations.

Think of it as a small safety buffer against any overestimations you might have made so far.

STEP 2: SET CALORIE TARGET

NOW THAT YOU HAVE ESTIMATED YOUR MAINTENANCE CALORIE INTAKE, YOU CAN MOVE ON TO SETTING YOUR FAT LOSS CALORIE TARGET.

Remember, you need to be in a state of negative calorie balance to shift your body into breakdown mode and to start mobilising body fat for use as fuel.

How Big Should the Calorie Deficit Be?

A key point to understand about calorie deficits is that the size of the deficit determines the rate of fat loss.

To help illustrate this we can use a meal planning rule of thumb called the '3,500 calorie rule'.

The rule is based on the premise that a single pound (0.45kg) of body fat contains roughly 3,500kcal. Therefore, if you create a 500kcal deficit each day, you will lose one pound (0.45kg) of body fat per week if your body only uses body fat to overcome the calorie deficit (3,500 / 500 = 7 days).

If you double the deficit size to 1,000kcal per day, you should theoretically lose two pounds (0.9kg) of body fat per week.

A key point to make here is that a bigger calorie deficit is not always better.

There is a limit to how quickly your body can mobilise body fat for use as fuel. Past a certain point, it will begin to break down and use muscle too.

While resistance training and eating a high-protein diet can help maintain or even increase muscle mass in a calorie deficit, research suggests that losing more than 1% of your total bodyweight per week increases the risk of muscle loss.

As a result, the aim throughout your transformation will be to lose on average 0.5-1% of your total bodyweight per week.

While there are advantages to the 'slow and steady' approach, we have set a lower limit of 0.5% as we are working to a fixed time frame and want to achieve the biggest possible change in your body composition.

Based on this, we can use the 3,500kcal rule to work out the size of calorie deficit required to achieve the target rate of bodyweight loss.

THERE IS A LIMIT TO HOW QUICKLY YOUR BODY CAN MOBILISE BODY FAT FOR USE AS FUEL. PAST A CERTAIN POINT, IT WILL BEGIN TO BREAK DOWN AND USE MUSCLE TOO.

WHILE RESISTANCE TRAINING AND EATING A HIGH-PROTEIN DIET CAN HELP MAINTAIN OR EVEN INCREASE MUSCLE MASS IN A CALORIE DEFICIT, RESEARCH SUGGESTS THAT LOSING MORE THAN 1% OF YOUR TOTAL BODYWEIGHT PER WEEK INCREASES THE RISK OF MUSCLE LOSS.

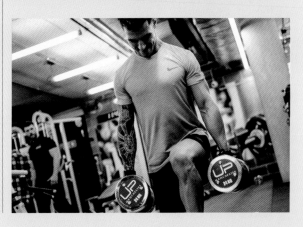

HOW TO CALCULATE YOUR CALORIE TARGET

STEP 1:
CALCULATE WEEKLY BODYWEIGHT LOSS TARGET

Although you could choose any value between 0.5-1%, we recommend using the mid-point, 0.75%, to calculate your initial nutrition targets.

STARTING BODYWEIGHT *(KG)*	X	0.75% *(in decimal form)*

To convert your weekly bodyweight loss target into decimal form you need to divide it by 100, so 0.75% becomes 0.0075.

STEP 2:
CALCULATE WEEKLY CALORIE DEFICIT

The 3,500kcal rule applies to pounds. To use kilograms, you need to multiply it by 2.2 and use 7,700 instead.

WEEKLY WEIGHT LOSS TARGET *(KG)*	X	7,700

STEP 3:
CALCULATE DAILY CALORIE DEFICIT

Divide your weekly calorie deficit by seven to spread it evenly across the week.

WEEKLY CALORIE DEFICIT ÷ 7

STEP 4:
CALCULATE DAILY CALORIE TARGET

To calculate your daily calorie target, subtract your daily calorie deficit from your estimated maintenance calorie intake.

ESTIMATED MAINTENANCE CALORIE INTAKE	–	DAILY CALORIE DEFICIT

How Accurate is the 3,500 Calorie Rule?

The 3,500kcal rule is a useful meal planning tool, but it is not foolproof.

Experience and research both show that fat loss very rarely occurs at the exact rate you plan for on paper. This is because:

▶ Your maintenance calorie intake is an estimate, so you cannot be completely sure what size of calorie deficit you are creating at the start.

▶ Your body makes adaptations when in a calorie deficit to conserve energy, which means that the same size calorie deficit will become progressively less effective over time.

There is also the added complication that bodyweight fluctuations caused by water retention can make it appear like you are losing body fat more slowly or quickly than you expect.

The key point is, like when selecting an activity multiplier, setting your initial calorie target is not an exact science.

The aim is to find a reasonable starting point that places you close to the target 0.5-1% bodyweight reduction per week. You can then make adjustments based on how your body responds over the course of your diet.

THE AIM IS TO FIND A REASONABLE STARTING POINT THAT PLACES YOU CLOSE TO THE TARGET 0.5-1% BODYWEIGHT REDUCTION PER WEEK. YOU CAN THEN MAKE ADJUSTMENTS BASED ON HOW YOUR BODY RESPONDS OVER THE COURSE OF YOUR DIET.

STEP 3: SET MACRONUTRIENT TARGETS

What Are Macronutrients?

Macronutrients are types of nutrients that your body needs in large amounts, and you may well be familiar with the three main types: protein, fat and carbohydrate.

On top of performing several other important roles, each macronutrient provides your body with a certain amount of energy:

Alcohol (ethanol) is also a source of energy and contains seven calories per gram. However, it is not essential to your survival or performance, and so we will not be setting a target intake.

Apart from certain confectionary items (which are pure carbohydrate) and oils (which are pure fat), most foods consist of at least two macronutrients.

You can calculate the calorie content of a food or drink by adding up the energy provided by each of the macronutrients it contains.

PROTEIN	FAT	CARBOHYDRATE
4KCAL PER GRAM	**9KCAL** PER GRAM	**4KCAL** PER GRAM

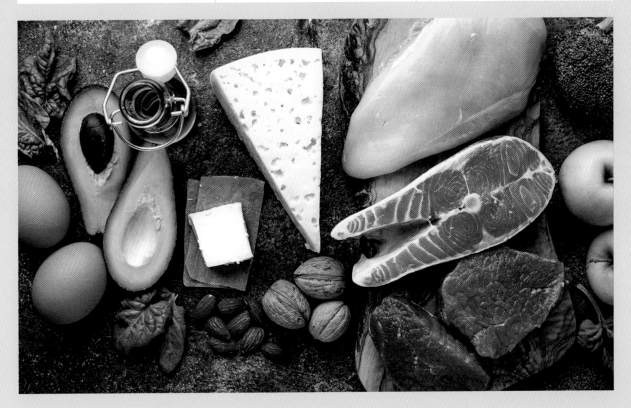

The Roles of Macronutrients

Each macronutrient plays a different role in the body and taking time to understand this will help you to set targets in the next section.

PROTEIN

The main role of protein in the body is structural, which means that your body uses it to build, maintain and replace substances like muscles, bones, connective tissue, hormones, enzymes, skin, hair and nails.

While not its primary role, protein is also a viable energy source and your body uses it to meet roughly 5% of your daily energy requirements under non-calorie restricted conditions.

Gram for gram, protein is the most satiating (filling) macronutrient, which can indirectly help fat loss by making it easier to stick to a calorie-restricted diet.

FAT

The main role of fat is to provide an energy source, a job it is well-equipped to perform. A single gram of fat provides 9kcal of energy, which is more than twice the amount available from an equivalent quantity of protein or carbohydrate.

Low-fat diets (think white fish and chicken) can be bland and boring. In contrast, fat-rich foods (think steak and nuts) add flavour and texture to your diet.

Dietary fat can help suppress hunger between meals, as it takes a relatively long time to digest and clear from your stomach. However, it is not an acute hunger suppressor (like protein and fibre-rich foods) and is very easy to overeat.

Dietary fat supports important biological functions, such as transporting fat-soluble vitamins (vitamin A, D, E and K) and hormone production (there is research linking very low-fat diets to decreases in testosterone levels - unfortunately, high-fat diets do not boost testosterone!).

Dietary fat provides two specific types of fatty acids, omega-3 and omega-6, which are essential nutrients. You require these for optimal health and must get them from your diet.

CARBOHYDRATE

Like fats, the main role of carbohydrates is to provide an energy source, especially during high-intensity exercise such as resistance training.

Unlike protein and fats, carbohydrates are not essential nutrients and you technically do not require any to survive. Nevertheless, many experts consider them to be 'conditionally essential' for maximising performance in high-intensity exercise.

In practical terms, aiming for 0g carbohydrate is unrealistic due to the small amounts contained in fat-rich foods, fruit and vegetables.

Like low-fat diets, low-carbohydrate diets can be restrictive in terms of food options and therefore difficult to sustain long-term.

A specific type of carbohydrate, fibre, is vital for digestive health and we will outline more specific fibre intake recommendations in the *Transformation Foods'* section.

HOW TO SET YOUR MACRONUTRIENT TARGETS

Protein Target

We set protein intake first as it is arguably the most important macronutrient for body composition, due to its ability to suppress hunger and build muscle.

Protein intake recommendations are set based on LBM, rather than total bodyweight. This makes sense given that body fat does not require large amounts of protein.

The recommended minimum protein intake for sedentary adults to prevent deficiency and negative health outcomes is 0.8 grams per kilogram of total bodyweight.

Most experts agree that this recommendation is outdated and that more protein is needed under certain conditions:

▶ When resistance training several times a week to help repair and replace damaged muscle.

▶ When following a calorie-restricted diet, your body becomes more reliant on protein as a source of energy. This reduces the amount available for muscle growth and repair, and increases the risk that your existing muscle mass will be sacrificed for use as fuel.

Researchers have so far failed to find any negative health outcomes for protein intakes of up to 3g per kilogram of total bodyweight in healthy individuals with no kidney-related issues - that's a lot of chicken!

However, it is unlikely that your muscles have a functional demand for this much protein and any extra benefit would be related to hunger-suppression or personal preference.

WE SET PROTEIN INTAKE FIRST AS IT IS ARGUABLY THE MOST IMPORTANT MACRONUTRIENT FOR BODY COMPOSITION, DUE TO ITS HUNGER-SUPPRESSING AND MUSCLE BUILDING ABILITY.

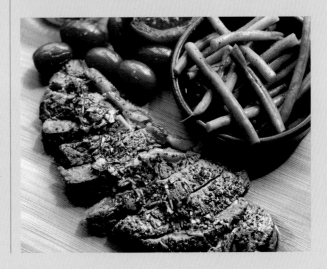

PROTEIN INTAKE RECOMMENDATIONS

Recommended lower limit for individuals who resistance train but struggle to eat a lot of protein	**2.0g per kg of LBM**
Recommended starting point for the average trainee	**2.4g per kg of LBM**
Recommended upper limit to leave enough calories for fat and carbohydrate	**2.8g per kg of LBM**

Note: You can select any value between 2.0 – 2.8g per kg of LBM

Fat and Carbohydrate Targets

Unlike protein, we prescribe fat and carbohydrate intake recommendations as a percentage of total calories.

The primary roles of fat and carbohydrate are to provide energy, so it makes sense to scale them to your total calorie (energy) intake.

We are addressing fats and carbohydrates together as the target you choose for one will determine your target for the other. As you can see in the tables below, we set fat first and then allocate any remaining calories to carbohydrate.

Research studies have repeatedly shown that fat loss will occur on any variation of fat to carbohydrate ratio if a calorie deficit is in place.

One way to help decide if you prefer fat, carbohydrate or have no real preference is to review the food tables in the 'Transformation Foods' section.

Because fat and carbohydrate intake is mostly a matter of personal preference, some people prefer to only track their protein and calorie intake. While this can work, we recommend setting specific targets to help with meal planning, but not overly worrying if some days you eat more carbohydrate and less fat, or vice-versa.

For more advice on how accurate you need to be when aiming for your fat and carbohydrate targets, refer to the 'Serving Size FAQs' section.

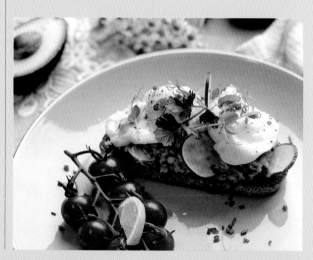

THE PRIMARY ROLES OF FAT AND CARBOHYDRATE ARE TO PROVIDE ENERGY, SO IT MAKES SENSE TO SCALE THEM TO YOUR TOTAL CALORIE (ENERGY) INTAKE.

FAT INTAKE RECOMMENDATIONS	
Recommended lower limit for individuals who prefer a higher carbohydrate (and lower fat) diet	25% of total calories
Recommended starting point for the average trainee	35% of total calories
Recommended upper limit for individuals who prefer a higher fat (and lower carbohydrate) diet	45% of total calories

Note: You can select any value between 25-45% of total calories

CARBOHYDRATE INTAKE RECOMMENDATIONS	
Allocate remaining calories to carbohydrates	Remaining calories

LBM = leem body mass.

HOW TO CALCULATE YOUR MACRONUTRIENT TARGETS

STEP 1:
CALCULATE PROTEIN TARGET

Select your protein multiplier from the protein intake recommendations table and apply it to your LBM in kilograms.

LBM (KG)	X	PROTEIN MULTIPLIER

STEP 2:
CALCULATE TOTAL PROTEIN CALORIES

Multiply your protein target by four to calculate how many calories you will consume from protein (you will see why in step 4).

PROTEIN TARGET	X	4

STEP 3:
CALCULATE FAT TARGET

Select your fat target from the fat intake recommendations table and multiply it by your calorie target.

CALORIE TARGET	X	FAT % TARGET (in decimal form)

To convert your fat target into decimal form you need to divide it by 100, so 35% becomes 0.35, 25% becomes 0.25, and so on.

Divide your answer by nine to calculate your fat target.

FAT CALORIES ÷ 9

STEP 4:
CALCULATE CARBOHYDRATE TARGET

Add your protein and fat calories together and subtract the answer from your daily calorie target. This will tell you how many calories you have left for carbohydrates.

CALORIE TARGET	_	(PROTEIN CALORIES + FAT CALORIES)

Divide your answer by four to calculate your carbohydrate target.

CARBOHYDRATE CALORIES ÷ 4

Once done, you should have targets for protein, fat and carbohydrate.

TRANSFORMATION NUMBER CASE STUDIES

TO HELP BRING THE TRANSFORMATION NUMBER THEORY TO LIFE WE WILL NOW FOLLOW
TWO EXAMPLE CLIENTS, ANDREW AND JENNY, THROUGH THE FULL SET-UP PROCESS.

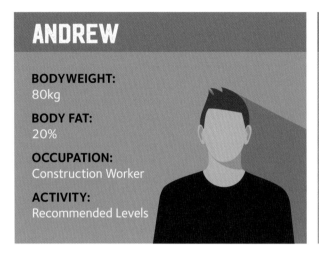

ANDREW

BODYWEIGHT:
80kg

BODY FAT:
20%

OCCUPATION:
Construction Worker

ACTIVITY:
Recommended Levels

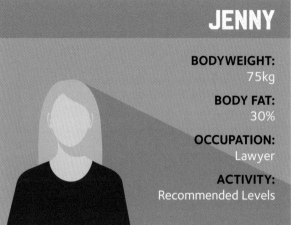

JENNY

BODYWEIGHT:
75kg

BODY FAT:
30%

OCCUPATION:
Lawyer

ACTIVITY:
Recommended Levels

STEP 1: ESTIMATE MAINTENANCE

Estimate RMR Using the Katch-McArdle Formula (p.34)

Example Calculations:

80kg x 0.2 (20% body fat)

= Andrew has 16kg of body fat.

80kg − 16kg

= Andrew has 64kg of LBM.

Katch McArdle Part 1: 21.6 x 64kg

= 1,382

Katch McArdle Part 2: = 1,382 + 370

= Andrew's RMR is 1,750kcal.

Example Calculations:

75kg x 0.3 (30% body fat)

= Jenny has 22.5kg of body fat.

75kg − 22.5kg

= Jenny has 52.5kg of LBM.

Katch McArdle Part 1: 21.6 x 52.5kg

= 1,134

Katch McArdle Part 2: = 1,134 + 370

= Jenny's RMR is 1,505kcal.

Note: Final values rounded to the nearest 5kcal.

Andrew has a physically demanding job and spends his working hours constantly on his feet. He also has to carry heavy objects around a construction site.

This makes hitting his daily step target easy.

He has committed to four resistance training workouts and one formal cardio workout per week.

Based on this, he chooses an activity multiplier of 'x 1.8'.

Example Calculations:

1,750kcal x 1.8

= **Andrew's estimated maintenance calorie intake is 3,150kcal.**

Note: Final values rounded to the nearest 5kcal.

Jenny has a sedentary job and spends several hours sat at her desk sending emails each day.

Hitting the minimum 10,000-daily step target is challenging, but she manages it by breaking up her day with short walks.

She has committed to three resistance training workouts and two formal cardio workouts per week.

Based on this, she chooses an activity multiplier of 'x 1.5'.

Example Calculations:

1,505kcal x 1.5

= **Jenny's estimated maintenance calorie intake is 2,255kcal.**

STEP 2: SET CALORIE TARGET

Example Calculations:

80kg x 0.0075 (0.75%)

= **Andrew's weekly bodyweight loss target is 0.6kg.**

0.6kg x 7,700kcal

= **Andrew's weekly calorie deficit is 4,620kcal.**

4,620kcal / 7

= **Andrew's daily calorie deficit is 660kcal.**

3,150kcal − 660kcal

= **Andrew's daily calorie target is 2,490kcal.**

Example Calculations:

75kg x 0.0075 (0.75%)

= **Jenny's weekly bodyweight loss target is 0.56kg.**

0.56kg x 7,700kcal

= **Jenny's weekly calorie deficit is 4,312kcal.**

4,312kcal / 7

= **Jenny's daily calorie deficit is 616kcal.**

2,255kcal − 616kcal

= **Jenny's daily calorie target is 1,640kcal.**

Note: Final values rounded to the nearest 5kcal.

STEP 3: SET MACRONUTRIENT TARGETS

Calculate Protein Target (p.41)

Andrew has a physically demanding job and trains several times per week.

He has also dieted before and likes how high-protein meals keep him feeling full.

Based on this, he chooses a protein multiplier of 'x 2.8'.

Example Calculations:

64kg x 2.8

180g x 4kcal

= **Andrew's protein target is 180g (720kcal).**

Jenny has only just started her fitness journey and never really focused on nutrition.

She knows that protein is important, but does not enjoy eating large servings of protein-rich foods.

Based on this, she chooses a protein multiplier of 'x 2'.

Example Calculations:

52.5kg x 2.0

105g x 4kcal

= **Jenny's protein target is 105g (420kcal).**

Calculate Fat Target (p.42)

Andrew typically feels best on a high-carbohydrate diet and starts to feel sluggish when his intake gets too low.

Based on this, he chooses a fat percentage target of 25%.

Example Calculations:

2,490kcal x 0.25 (25%)

= **Andrew consumes 623kcal from fat per day.**

623kcal / 9kcal

= **Andrew's fat target is 70g.**

Jenny has always read that carbohydrates make you fat, but has now learned that controlling calories is the most important factor.

Based on this, she chooses a fat percentage target of 35%.

Example Calculations:

1,640kcal x 0.35 (35%)

= **Jenny consumes 574kcal from fat per day.**

574kcal / 9kcal

= **Jenny's fat target is 65g.**

Calculate Carbohydrate Target (p.42)

Example Calculations:

2,490kcal – (720kcal + 623kcal)

= **Andrew's daily calorie intake from carbohydrate is 1,147kcal.**

1,147kcal / 4kcal

= **Andrew's carbohydrate target is 285g.**

Example Calculations:

1,640kcal – (420kcal + 574kcal)

= **Jenny's daily calorie intake from carbohydrate is 646kcal.**

646kcal / 4

= **Jenny's carbohydrate target is 160g.**

FINAL TRANSFORMATION NUMBERS

Protein: 180g	Protein: 105g
Fat: 70g	Fat: 65g
Carbohydrate: 285g	Carbohydrate: 160g
Calories:2,490kcal	Calories:1,640kcal

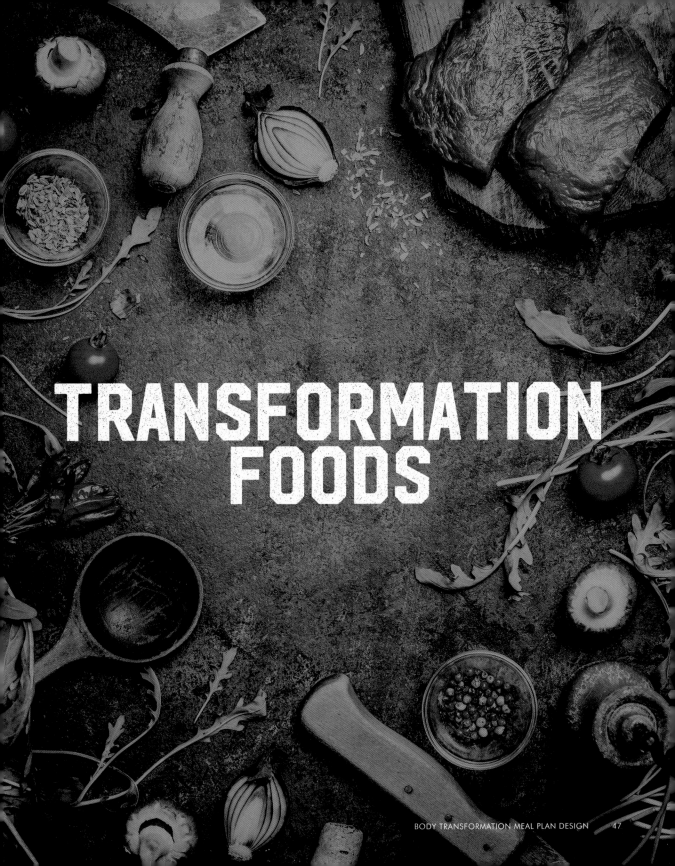

TRANSFORMATION FOODS

TRANSFORMATION FOODS

NOW THAT YOU HAVE SET UP FOR SUCCESS, THE NEXT STEP IS TO CALCULATE THE NUTRITION TARGETS THAT YOU WILL USE TO CREATE YOUR MEAL PLAN.

Before continuing, there are some key points we need to address.

KEY POINT 1 — THERE IS NO SUCH THING AS A 'FAT LOSS FOOD'

WHILE IT IS TRUE THAT STANDARD SERVINGS OF SOME FOODS CONTAIN VERY FEW CALORIES, THE IDEA OF A 'NEGATIVE-CALORIE' FOOD IS A MYTH.

For this to be the case, the thermic effect of food (TEF) would have to be more than 100%, meaning that the caloric cost of digesting the food is greater than its actual energy content.

Protein has the highest TEF of all nutrients at 20-30%, which still leaves at least 70% of the calories for your body to use or store.

All foods add at least some calories to your calorie balance - no foods subtract them.

Overeating any type of food, even those labelled as 'healthy', will lead to weight gain.

KEY POINT 2 — THERE IS NO SUCH THING AS A 'FATTENING FOOD'

PART OF DEVELOPING A HEALTHY RELATIONSHIP WITH FOOD IS UNDERSTANDING THAT NO FOOD IS NATURALLY 'BAD' FOR YOU.

In terms of 'weight loss', a calorie is a calorie and if you are in a state of negative calorie balance, you can technically eat anything you want and still lose weight.

But, if you are interested in losing body fat and building muscle, then you should not interpret this as being a free license to eat whatever you want.

BUT, IF YOU ARE INTERESTED IN LOSING BODY FAT AND BUILDING MUSCLE, THEN YOU SHOULD NOT INTERPRET THIS AS BEING A FREE LICENSE TO EAT WHATEVER YOU WANT.

FOODS THAT ARE GOOD FOR FAT LOSS SHARE ONE OR MORE OF THE FOLLOWING CHARACTERISTICS:

1. Contain few calories per gram.
2. Solid, rather than liquid composition.
3. High in fibre.
4. High in protein.

Examples include whole and minimally processed foods (close to their natural form) like fresh fruit, vegetables and meats.

These types of food are also typically nutrient-dense and provide several micronutrients that have positive health effects.

While we would never recommend completely removing a specific food from your diet (unless medically advised to do so), limiting your intake of certain foods can make it easier to stick to your meal plan.

These foods are basically the opposite of those mentioned before. Examples include obvious things like alcohol, sodas, sweets and fast-foods, but you also must be careful with certain 'healthy' foods like nuts and oils (fat loss does not necessarily follow healthy eating, and vice-versa).

Everybody also has their own personal 'trigger foods' that they struggle to eat only in moderation.

CALORIE DENSITY OF FOOD

EXAMPLE OF 500 KCAL PORTIONS

LIQUID CALORIES	HEAVILY PROCESSED FOODS	LEAN PROTEINS	FRUITS & VEGETABLES

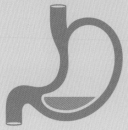 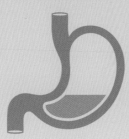 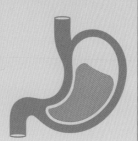 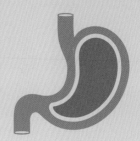

We typically recommend limiting consumption of calorie-dense foods, which are those that contain a high number of calories per unit of volume.

The problem with calorie-dense foods is that while eating a large proportion of your calories in one sitting may taste great in the moment; it can cause big fluctuations in your energy levels and leave you feeling hungry later in the day.

For example, you could very easily eat 500kcal worth of pizza and be hungry soon after. In contrast, a calorie-equated serving of lean protein and vegetables would keep you full for hours.

YOUR SHOPPING LIST

Before starting your transformation challenge, we recommend performing an inventory of your fridge and kitchen cupboards.

Start by ditching any 'non diet-friendly' foods (preferably by donating them to charity rather than having one last hurrah). You are more likely to make bad food choices if you have tempting foods in your kitchen.

The next step is to stock up on the ingredients that will be the staples of your new diet.

To keep things simple, we have grouped foods based on whether they will help to hit your protein, fat or carbohydrate target.

Although detailed, the food tables are not a complete database of every known food and drink. Instead, they are the choices that we believe are most conducive to fat loss, staying healthy and what we recommend basing most of your diet around.

START BY DITCHING ANY 'NON DIET-FRIENDLY' FOODS (PREFERABLY BY DONATING THEM TO CHARITY RATHER THAN HAVING ONE LAST HURRAH). YOU ARE MORE LIKELY TO MAKE BAD FOOD CHOICES IF YOU HAVE TEMPTING FOODS IN YOUR KITCHEN.

PROTEIN

PROTEIN SOURCES		
SOURCE	**LEAN PROTEIN**	**FATTY PROTEIN**
MEAT	Lean beef	Beef steak – sirloin, fillet, ribeye
	Lean minced meat (turkey, chicken, beef)	Duck
	Lean pork	Fatty minced meat (beef, lamb, pork)
	Venison	Lamb
		Pork
FISH	Cod	Mackerel
	Haddock	Salmon
	King prawns	Seabass
	Tuna (canned in brine or spring water)	Smoked salmon
	Tuna steak	Trout
POULTRY	Chicken breast	Chicken leg/thigh
	Turkey breast	
OTHER	Egg whites	Whole eggs
	Greek yoghurt	
	Protein powders	

Animal vs Plant Protein Sources

The two main types of protein source are:

▶ **Animal-origin:** meat, fish, poultry, eggs and dairy.

▶ **Plant-origin:** soy-based products, grains, nuts, seeds and legumes.

Proteins consist of smaller sub-units called amino acids. There are 20 different amino acids in the food supply, nine of which are 'essential amino acids' (EAAs), which means that you must get them from your diet.

The EAA content of a protein source is the primary determinant of its quality. Every meal does not have to include all the EAAs, but you do need to get enough of each type over the course of a whole day for the best muscle building results.

Animal-origin protein sources contain all the EAAs your body needs and are 'complete' proteins. In contrast, many (but not all) plant sources are deficient in one or more and are 'incomplete'.

Meat eaters do not have to worry about their EAA intake if they meet their daily protein target, but plant-based dieters need to be more strategic with their meal planning.

Advice to Plant-Based Dieters

The biggest challenge you will face is getting enough protein while controlling your overall calorie intake. For example, whereas protein accounts for 80% of the total calories in a 150g sirloin steak, it only makes up 35% of an equivalent number of calories from almonds.

If only a small percentage of a food's total calorie content comes from the target macronutrient (in this case, protein), then you must consume larger servings and therefore more calories to meet your target.

The table below lists some of the lowest calorie plant-origin protein sources. Specifically, it shows the serving size required for 20g protein and how many calories this equates to.

We recommend consuming at least part of your daily protein intake in supplement form. Most health food stores also offer a varied selection of organic whole food meat alternatives.

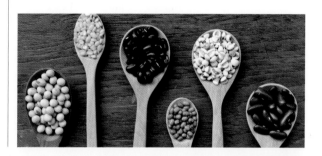

LOW-CALORIE PLANT-ORIGIN PROTEIN SOURCES
Serving sizes and calories required for 20g protein

SOURCE	UNCOOKED SERVING	CALORIES
Vegan protein powders (generic)	30g	100kcal
Tofu	155g	185kcal
Soya beans (drained)	145g	200kcal
Tempeh	105g	222kcal
Pinto beans (drained)	285g	255kcal
Edamame	145g	265kcal
Black beans (drained)	285g	275kcal
Kidney beans (drained)	285g	310kcal

Lean and Fatty Protein Sources

We have categorised animal-origin protein sources as either 'lean' or 'fatty':

▶ Lean protein sources contain less than 10% fat per 100g of uncooked weight.

▶ Fatty protein sources contain more than 10% fat per 100g of uncooked weight.

The table below shows how easy it is to consume extra calories while eating equivalent servings of a lean and fatty protein source.

Including more lean than fatty protein sources in your diet will leave you with more calories left over after hitting your protein target. This will allow you to include a greater volume of foods elsewhere in your diet, which is key to staying full.

Fatty protein sources are not unhealthy. In fact, fatty fish like salmon and mackerel are key sources of essential fatty acids, and red meats like steak contain several important micronutrients, such as B vitamins, zinc and iron.

We have listed the most common lean and fatty protein sources, but be aware that the caloric content of a protein source can vary based on several factors:

▶ The specific 'cut', e.g. fillet vs ribeye steak.

▶ Processing method, e.g. minced meat can range from 5-30% fat based on the type of meat used.

▶ Several fatty protein sources are now available in reduced fat versions.

▶ Differences between suppliers for the same type of product.

PROTEIN SOURCE	UNCOOKED SERVING	CALORIES	PROTEIN	FAT
Cod Fillet	100g	80kcal	90%	10%
Salmon Fillet	100g	200kcal	50%	55%

Protein Supplements

Protein powders can be a convenient source of protein when you are:

▶ Unable to prepare a meal, e.g. when travelling.

▶ Short of time, e.g. between work meetings.

▶ Struggling with appetite, e.g. early in the morning.

Liquid meals are not as filling as whole food meals, but you can bulk out your shake with fruit and vegetables, or combine powders with other foods like yoghurt and oats to make a more satisfying meal.

Protein powders are also available as food bars, which typically provide around 20g protein per bar. Protein bars can help satisfy cravings for sweet foods, but they are relatively calorie-dense and quick to eat.

WE RECOMMEND LIMITING PROTEIN SUPPLEMENTS TO 20% OF YOUR DAILY PROTEIN INTAKE AND USING WHOLE FOOD SOURCES TO MEET THE REST OF YOUR TARGET. FOR MOST PEOPLE, THIS WILL EQUATE TO ONE PROTEIN SHAKE PER DAY.

Watch out for 'mass gainer' protein powders that are typically low in quality, but high in calories. Select a product that has less than 5g carbohydrate per 100g (vegan protein powders may contain more than 5g).

We recommend limiting protein supplements to 20% of your daily protein intake and using whole food sources to meet the rest of your target. For most people, this will equate to one protein shake per day.

EXTRA CONSIDERATIONS

Certain fish such as swordfish and tuna contain high levels of mercury. Eating lots of these fish (several times per week for prolonged periods) causes mercury to build up in your body to potentially dangerous levels. Best practice is to limit intake to one to two portions per week.

You can add variety to your protein intake by trying out game and exotic cuts of meat that are now more readily available in butchers and supermarkets.

FAT

TYPE	SOURCE	SFA (%)	MUFA (%)	PUFA (%)
	FAT SOURCES			
NUTS	Almonds	8%	66%	26%
	Brazil nuts	25%	41%	34%
	Cashews	20%	60%	20%
	Hazelnuts	8%	78%	14%
	Pecans	9%	59%	31%
	Walnuts	6%	28%	66%
	Nut butters (all types)	10%	68%	22%
SEEDS	Chia seeds	11%	7%	81%
	Flaxseeds	9%	19%	72%
	Sesame seeds	15%	39%	46%
	Sunflower seeds	10%	40%	50%
BUTTERS AND OILS	Butter	68%	28%	4%
	Coconut oil	92%	6%	2%
	Olive oil	14%	75%	11%
DAIRY	Cheddar cheese	67%	30%	3%
	Dark chocolate (70%+)	63%	33%	3%
	Feta cheese	74%	23%	3%
	Goats cheese	73%	24%	3%
	Mozzarella cheese	64%	32%	4%
	Parmesan cheese	64%	31%	4%
OTHER	Avocado	15%	72%	13%
	Fatty protein sources	–	–	–
	Whole eggs	37%	46%	17%

Know Your Fats: Good and Bad

There are three main types of dietary fat, which all have different chemical structures and effects on your body: saturated fatty acids (SFAs), monounsaturated fatty acids (MUFAs) and polyunsaturated fatty acids (PUFAs).

Most fat-rich foods contain a mix of all three but are typically higher in one type, which determines their physical properties. Fat sources proportionately higher in SFAs are solid at room temperature, whereas those higher in unsaturated fats tend to be softer (or liquid).

Saturated Fat (SFA)

Fat sources high in SFAs include animal products like meat, egg yolks and dairy fats. Coconut oil is one of the few plant sources high in SFAs.

SFAs have a bad reputation, and some research studies have associated high intakes with an increased risk of heart disease. However, if you exercise regularly, control your calorie intake and include a balance of fats in your diet, then the risks are minimal.

Completely removing SFAs from your diet would be very difficult and require extreme dietary changes that would most likely result in an insufficient protein intake and several micronutrient deficiencies.

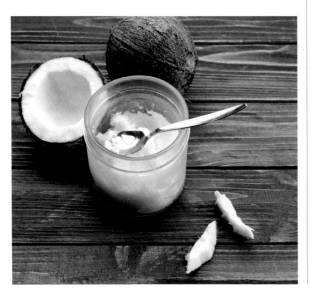

Monounsaturated Fat (MUFA)

Fat sources high in MUFAs include various meats, olive oil and the oil in avocados, nuts and seeds.

Most health organisations label MUFAs as 'healthy fats' and research suggests that they may help lower levels of LDL (bad) cholesterol.

MUFAs will make up most of your total fat intake, as sources like nuts and oils are easy to add to your meals.

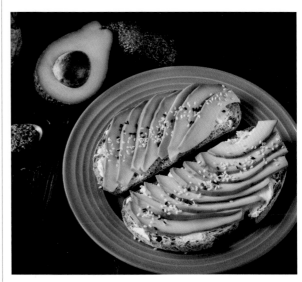

Polyunsaturated Fat (PUFA)

The two main types of PUFAs are omega-3 and omega-6. Unlike other fats, they are essential nutrients, and you must include them as part of your diet.

Most people naturally consume enough omega-6, but it is a lot more common for people to get suboptimal amounts of omega-3.

Research on the positive health effects of omega-3 mostly focuses on two specific types, eicosapentaenoic acid (EPA) and docosahexaenoic acid (DHA), which are collectively known as fish oils.

Fish oils have wide-ranging effects on the body and can help reduce the risk of heart disease, stroke, diabetes and several other negative health outcomes.

Most of the beneficial effects of fish oil occur over a period of weeks and months. Therefore, it is better to think of it as a nutritional insurance policy rather than a 'magic bullet'.

Fatty fish, such as salmon and mackerel, are the best sources and we recommend including them as protein sources in your meal plan two to three times per week.

Plant sources, such as flaxseed and walnuts, contain a type of omega-3, called alpha-linolenic acid (ALA), which converts to EPA and DHA in the body. However, the conversion process is not very efficient, and we recommend focusing on marine sources for the greatest benefit.

Fish oil supplements can help simplify your meal planning and are a viable alternative for vegetarians and anyone who does not like the taste of fish.

For more information on optimal fish oil supplementation dosage turn to the *'Supplements'* section.

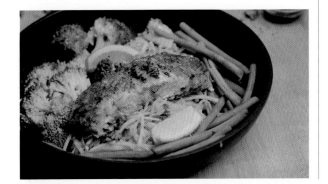

'Bad Fats' – Trans Fatty Acids (TFAs)

TFAs are man-made artificial fats found almost exclusively in processed foods to extend their shelf life. Examples include cakes, biscuits, ready meals and fast-foods.

TFAs have no associated health benefits, and you should keep your intake to a minimum. Look out for the terms 'partially hydrogenated' and 'trans fatty acids' on nutrition labels to spot foods containing them.

When eating a diet based on whole and minimally processed foods, you do not need to worry about consuming too many TFAs.

Most companies are reformulating their products to reduce or eliminate TFAs now that they must declare TFA content on nutrition labels.

TFAS HAVE NO ASSOCIATED HEALTH BENEFITS, AND YOU SHOULD KEEP YOUR INTAKE TO A MINIMUM. LOOK OUT FOR THE TERMS 'PARTIALLY HYDROGENATED' AND 'TRANS FATTY ACIDS' ON NUTRITION LABELS TO SPOT FOODS CONTAINING THEM.

EXTRA CONSIDERATIONS

Fat is the most calorie-dense macronutrient and therefore easy to overeat. We strongly recommend paying close attention to nutrition labels and using digital food scales to measure your serving sizes where possible.

A primary use of oils is to prevent sticking during the cooking process. To free up extra calories to use elsewhere in your diet, try cooking with non-stick pans or a minimal amount of low-calorie cooking spray.

CARBOHYDRATE

CARBOHYDRATE SOURCES		
NON-STARCHY VEGETABLES	**FRUIT**	**STARCHY VEGETABLES / GRAINS**
Asparagus	Apple	Beans (all types)
Beetroot	Banana	Brown rice
Broccoli	Blackberries	Couscous
Brussels sprouts	Blueberries	Oatmeal (all types)
Cabbage	Grapefruit	Parsnip
Carrots	Kiwifruit	Quinoa
Cauliflower	Orange	Sweet potato
Celery	Pineapple	Wild rice
Courgette	Raspberries	White potato
Green beans	Strawberries	Whole grain products
Kale	Watermelon	
Lettuce		
Mushrooms		
Onions		
Peppers		
Rocket		
Spinach		
Tomatoes		
Watercress		

The three main types of carbohydrate are simple sugars, starch and fibre, which you will find in varying amounts in our recommended carbohydrate sources: vegetables, fruits and grains.

Vegetables: Starchy vs Non-Starchy

Vegetables are packed full of micronutrients and are your main source of dietary fibre.

Vegetables can be classified as either starchy or non-starchy based on their carbohydrate content:

► Non-starchy vegetables contain less than 10g carbohydrate per 100g of uncooked weight.

► Starchy-vegetables contain more than 10g carbohydrate per 100g of uncooked weight.

Non-starchy vegetables are a dieter's secret weapon, as they contain very few calories per serving. One of the first recommendations we give to clients struggling with hunger is to add more non-starchy vegetables to their meal plan.

STARCHY VEGETABLES ARE ALSO A GREAT SOURCE OF MICRONUTRIENTS AND FIBRE BUT ARE MORE CALORIE-DENSE AND THEREFORE YOU MUST PAY CLOSE ATTENTION TO YOUR SERVING SIZES. FOR EXAMPLE, IT WOULD BE ALMOST IMPOSSIBLE TO OVEREAT ON KALE, BUT YOU CAN VERY EASILY CONSUME A LARGE NUMBER OF CALORIES EATING POTATOES.

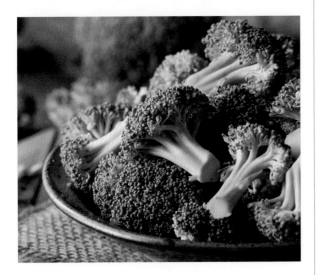

Starchy vegetables are also a great source of micronutrients and fibre but are more calorie-dense and therefore you must pay close attention to your serving sizes. For example, it would be almost impossible to overeat on kale, but you can very easily consume a large number of calories eating potatoes.

As a result, we have listed starchy vegetables alongside grains in the food tables as they are more similar in calorie content.

The nutrient content of vegetables can deteriorate during cooking. For example, boiling vegetables for too long can cause the nutrients to leach into the water. Try steaming or stir-frying them instead and include a mixture of raw and cooked types in your diet.

Fruit: Natural vs Refined Sugar

One of the main reasons people tend to avoid fruit is because of concerns over its sugar content and the impact this may have on their health.

An important distinction to make here is between natural food sources of sugar, like fruit, and refined sources, such as non-diet soft drinks, cakes and sweets.

While the sugar molecules found in fruit are chemically identical to those found in refined sugars, they also come packaged alongside a host of vitamins, minerals, fibre and other key nutrients.

Consider the example of an orange, which provides around 15g of carbohydrate, but also 12% of your daily fibre requirements, and nearly all the recommended amount of vitamin C.

In comparison, a tablespoon of table sugar contains an equivalent amount of carbohydrate, but nothing else. As a result, it is an example of 'empty calories' in that it provides energy, but little or no nutritional value.

Fruits make a great snack option, because:

▶ The high water and fibre content of most fruits mean that they contain relatively few calories per serving. For example, an average sized apple or banana both only contain roughly 100kcal.

▶ The naturally sweet flavour can help satisfy sugar cravings. Fructose, the primary carbohydrate in fruits, is the sweetest tasting sugar molecule and a key ingredient in food sweeteners.

Not all fruits are diet-friendly, and we do not recommend including dried fruits and fruit juices as staples in your transformation diet.

Dried fruits are more calorie-dense due to the removal of the water content and therefore easy to overeat. For example, 100g of grapes contains roughly 65kcal, whereas an equivalent serving size of raisins (dried grapes) contains 300kcal.

Fruit juices, like most liquid calories, are calorie-dense, digest very quickly, and do not send fullness signals to your brain.

Grains: Whole vs Refined

Unless your carbohydrate target is very low, you will struggle to get enough carbohydrates in your diet by only eating fruit and non-starchy vegetables. Including starchy vegetables and grains can help you to meet your target as they provide a more concentrated source of carbohydrates.

Any food made from cereal grains like wheat, rice and oats are grain products. There are two main types: refined grains and whole grains.

Refined grains have been processed to remove two thirds of the grain kernel (bran and germ) for a finer texture and longer shelf life. This also removes fibre, iron and many B vitamins. To account for this, most refined grains are 'enriched', which adds back some of the B vitamins and iron, but not the fibre. Common examples include breakfast cereals and white bread.

Whole grains contain the entire grain kernel and are also high in fibre and micronutrients. Common examples include oatmeal and brown rice.

If you control your calorie intake and make sure that refined grains do not displace more nutrient-dense foods in your diet, then you can include them without any adverse health effects.

However, we recommend prioritising whole grains as they are typically less calorie-dense and provide an additional source of micronutrients and fibre in your diet.

IF YOU CONTROL YOUR CALORIE INTAKE AND MAKE SURE THAT REFINED GRAINS DO NOT DISPLACE MORE NUTRIENT-DENSE FOODS IN YOUR DIET, THEN YOU CAN INCLUDE THEM WITHOUT ANY ADVERSE HEALTH EFFECTS.

Dietary Fibre

There are several different types of fibre, which can be divided into:

▶ **Soluble fibre:** dissolves in water and forms a thick gel-like substance in your digestive system.

▶ **Insoluble fibre:** does not dissolve in water and passes through your digestive system relatively intact.

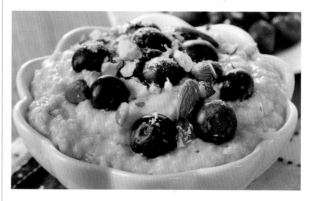

Soluble fibre slows down the digestive process by delaying gastric (stomach) emptying. This promotes a feeling of fullness and helps to control your blood sugar levels following a carbohydrate-rich meal.

Insoluble fibre has the opposite effect and works to speed up the digestive process by pushing foods through your system. This natural laxative effect helps to keep you 'regular' and is why many people refer to fibre as 'nature's broom'.

Including a balance of both types in your diet is important for digestive health and appetite control. They are typically found together in food sources such as fruits, vegetables and whole grain products.

You do not need to track your fibre intake if you include a variety of fruits, vegetables and whole grains in your diet.

A general recommendation is 15g per 1,000kcal, and at least 20g per day.

It is possible to consume too much fibre which can cause gastrointestinal discomfort and malabsorption of vitamins and minerals.

DRINKS AND CONDIMENTS

DRINKS AND CONDIMENTS	
DRINKS	**CONDIMENTS**
Water (still or sparkling)	Sea salt
Black coffee	Black pepper
Green tea	Herbs, seasonings & spices
Fruit and herbal teas	
Diet soda	

Fluid Intake

We all know that staying properly hydrated is extremely important. Symptoms of dehydration include headaches, irritability and impaired cognitive function and exercise performance.

Consuming fluids can also help with fat loss. Drinking a glass of water or other fluids before a meal has a filling effect which reduces the chances of overeating.

No fluid intake formula or guideline fits everyone perfectly. Hydration status is very individual and affected by factors such as the climate you live in and how much exercise you perform.

We recommend aiming for at least two litres per day and sticking to the following hydration habits:

▶ Fill up a big bottle of water (1-2 litres) and make it your goal to drink it each day.

▶ Drink a portion of this when you wake up (after weighing yourself) and then with every meal.

▶ Drink before, during and after exercise to replace water loss from sweating.

▶ All fluids, including coffee and tea, count towards your total. The only exception is alcohol, which has a purely dehydrating effect.

Caffeine Intake

The most common sources of caffeine are coffee, tea, sodas, energy drinks and pre-workout supplements.

In 2015, the European Food Safety Authority (EFSA) published a report advising that consuming up to 400mg per day from all sources does not raise safety concerns in healthy adults.

To help put this in context, we have compiled a table showing the caffeine content of some popular products.

CAFFEINE CONTENT

DRINK	Amount
Starbucks® Black Americano - Venti (L)	300mg
Starbucks® Black Americano - Grande (M)	225mg
Starbucks® Black Americano - Tall (S)	150mg
Red Bull® (250ml can)	80mg
Monster® (473ml can)	160mg
Instant Coffee (1 rounded teaspoon)	60mg
Diet Coke® (330ml can)	40mg
Pre-workout (Generic product)	200mg
Tea Leaves or Bags (150ml)	35mg

It is important to note that 400mg per day is a general guideline and people who are 'hypersensitive' to caffeine can experience negative symptoms from as little as 100mg per day.

IT IS IMPORTANT TO NOTE THAT 400MG PER DAY IS A GENERAL GUIDELINE AND PEOPLE WHO ARE 'HYPERSENSITIVE' TO CAFFEINE CAN EXPERIENCE NEGATIVE SYMPTOMS FROM AS LITTLE AS 100MG PER DAY.

When consumed in moderation, caffeine has the potential to improve your health, physical and mental performance. To get maximum benefit from your caffeine intake we recommend:

▶ Use the minimum effective dose.

▶ Consider only using it when you really need a functional boost, e.g. before a long drive or challenging workout.

▶ Schedule regular caffeine breaks, e.g. caffeine-free weekends, holidays or every few weeks.

▶ Exercise regularly and eat healthily to boost your energy levels naturally, e.g. taking walks or having a piece of fruit rather than relying on caffeine.

▶ Avoid caffeine from the early afternoon (2-3pm) onwards as it takes several hours to clear from your system.

Artificial Sweeteners and Diet Soda

Artificial sweeteners are calorie-free chemical substances that food manufacturers use instead of sugar to sweeten foods and drinks. They are a key ingredient in diet sodas and have received a large amount of attention (both positive and negative) from researchers and in the media.

The primary concerns are that they may have adverse health effects and trigger sugar cravings that cause you to overeat.

All artificial sweeteners undergo a rigorous safety assessment before manufacturers can include them in their products. There is also no evidence to suggest any long-term health risks from drinking diet soda.

Including diet sodas in your meal plan may help, rather than hinder, fat loss if it reduces your consumption of calorie-containing drinks like soda, fruit juices and alcohol.

One issue to be aware of is that most diet sodas contain caffeine which can be an issue if consumed in excess.

You do not have to include diet sodas in your meal plan but should not feel guilty about doing so in moderation either.

Excessive consumption of diet sodas (and low-calorie diet foods in general) can be a red flag for a negative relationship with food or an overly aggressive diet.

INCLUDING DIET SODAS IN YOUR MEAL PLAN MAY HELP, RATHER THAN HINDER, FAT LOSS IF IT REDUCES YOUR CONSUMPTION OF CALORIE-CONTAINING DRINKS LIKE SODA, FRUIT JUICES AND ALCOHOL.

ONE ISSUE TO BE AWARE OF IS THAT MOST DIET SODAS CONTAIN CAFFEINE WHICH CAN BE AN ISSUE IF CONSUMED IN EXCESS.

Alcohol

Alcohol (ethanol) is not an essential nutrient, which means that you do not need to include any in your diet.

In fact, many of our clients use the transformation period to 'detox' from alcohol completely.

Regarding alcohol and fat loss, potential issues to be aware of are:

▶ Alcohol is a form of liquid calories, which digest very quickly and do not send fullness signals to your brain.

▶ Drinking to the point of intoxication can impair impulse control and increase the chances of overeating.

▶ When consumed in excess, alcohol calories can displace other key nutrients in your diet.

However, there is no evidence to suggest that moderate alcohol consumption can directly impair fat loss if you control your calorie intake and have enough calories left for the required amounts of protein, fats and carbohydrates.

There is no set definition for moderation, but a simple guideline to follow during your transformation is to limit your intake to 10-15% of your daily calorie target one to two times per week.

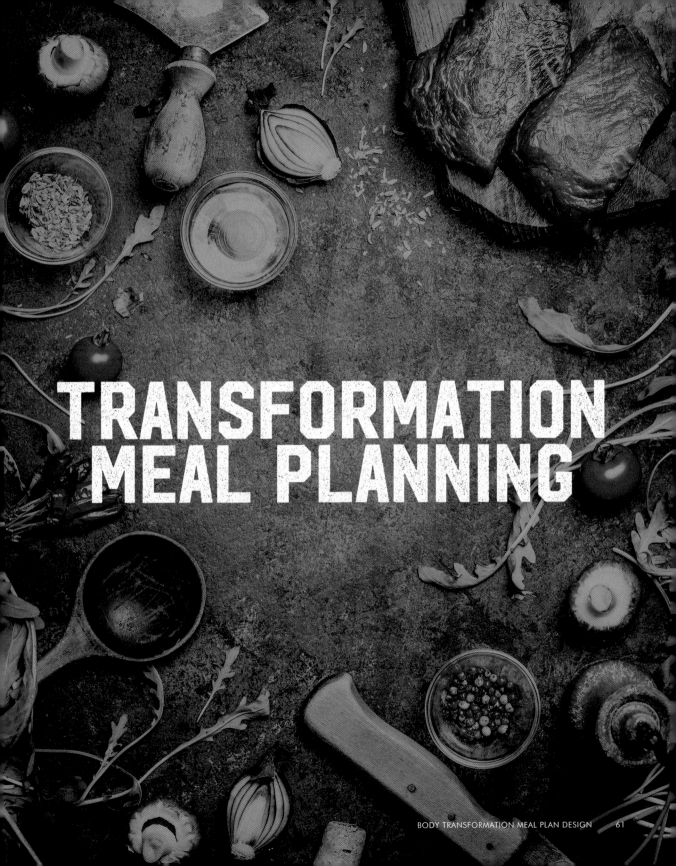

TRANSFORMATION MEAL PLANNING

TRANSFORMATION MEAL PLANNING

A MEAL PLAN IS AN ACTION PLAN FOR HOW TO APPROACH YOUR DIET FOR A SPECIFIC PERIOD, TYPICALLY ONE WEEK.

Admittedly, talking about the intricacies of meal planning is not as glamorous as discussing how to optimise your nutrition targets for muscle growth and fat loss, but it is just as important.

Without a meal plan, there are several scenarios that can crop up over the course of a transformation that have the potential to derail your progress. For example, you may find yourself:

▶ Travelling all day and only having access to airline or service station food.

▶ Eating in a restaurant with no diet-friendly options.

▶ Starving hungry and having to eat something.

These all sound like legitimate excuses for making less-than-optimal diet choices. However, the truth is that any slip-ups these events may cause are completely avoidable with a meal plan.

Travelling with limited access to food becomes a lot easier (and more cost effective) when you have pre-prepared your meals for the journey.

Likewise, searching for restaurants where you know that you can eat healthily makes dining out a lot less stressful of an experience.

And a combination of more regular eating patterns and portion control will help you to better manage your energy and hunger levels throughout the day.

MEAL PLANNNG ESSENTIALS

Digital Food Scales

Food scales will help you to hit your nutrition targets with a high degree of accuracy and provide a valuable education in serving sizes.

We recommend digital (rather than old-school analogue) scales for accuracy.

For advice on what foods you do and do not need to weigh, refer to the serving size FAQs.

Nutrition Tracking Application

Nutrition tracking applications are electronic food databases and food diaries that make it incredibly easy to write a meal plan. Specifically, you will use them to:

▶ Research the nutrition values of different foods.

▶ Calculate appropriate serving sizes.

▶ Keep a detailed record of your food intake.

There are several different applications to choose from, but we recommend MyFitnessPal (MFP), which you can download and use on your computer and smartphone.

HOW TO SET UP AND USE MYFITNESSPAL

We cannot provide a step-by-step set-up guide as it will become outdated as soon as MFP releases an update.

However, there are some key topics we need to address that should always be relevant and apply to all nutrition tracking applications.

Note: If you do want a more detailed user guide, you can find one on the MFP website, www.myfitnesspal.com.

Setting Nutrition Goals

The MFP goal setting feature makes it easy to track progress towards your daily nutrition targets. For example, how much more protein you need and the number of calories you have remaining.

By the way, MFP will try to suggest nutrition targets for you to follow. Ignore these and use the macronutrient and calorie targets you calculated earlier when setting up your profile.

Searching for Foods and Drinks

The MFP database is partly crowdsourced (entered by users). As a result, you will most likely find several entries for a single product (which often conflict), and some of them will contain errors.

There are three main ways to search the MFP database, which we have outlined below:

OPTION 1: MANUAL SEARCH	OPTION 2: BARCODE SCANNING	OPTION 3: RECENT ITEMS
1. Type the item's name into the search bar. 2. Select the most appropriate option from the search results.	1. Check if the item has a barcode. 2. Hover your smartphone's camera over the barcode. 3. MFP will automatically load the nutrition profile for you.	MFP allows you to save and remembers meals that you eat on a regular basis. (So, logging your meals will become easier over time).

Where possible, we recommend using the barcode scanning feature.

However, if you do perform a manual search, make sure to include the brand and full product name in your search. For example, 'Sainsbury's skinless chicken breast' rather than 'chicken breast' and 'Tesco sweet potato' rather than 'sweet potato'.

If you are eating mainly whole and minimally processed foods, then you should not have to worry too much about database errors.

For advice on how to track foods without nutrition labels, refer to the serving size FAQs.

SERVING SIZE FAQS

Q1 : DO I NEED TO HIT MY NUTRITION TARGETS TO THE GRAM?

QUICK ANSWER:
Aim to meet your calorie target within +/-50kcal and your protein target within a +/- 10g range. Do not worry if you miss your fat and carbohydrate targets.

Why?

Although you have calculated specific macronutrient targets, e.g. 155g protein, 60g fat and 100g carbohydrate, it is important to realise that it is not always possible, or expected, to meet these to the gram.

Instead, it is better to think of each target as a range where a small amount of variation above or below your target is acceptable.

The human body is remarkably resilient, and you will not lose muscle or develop a nutrient deficiency if you deviate from your targets for one day (but consistently missing your targets can cause problems).

The most important targets to aim for with a high degree of accuracy are your calorie and protein targets.

▶ Aim to meet your calorie target within a +/- 50kcal range. For example, if your calorie target is 2,000kcal, aim for between 1,950-2,050kcal.

▶ Aim to meet your protein target within a +/- 10g range. For example, if your target is 150g, aim for between 140-160g.

If you meet your protein target, but are below your calorie target and do not feel hungry, you do not need to 'eat up' to your calorie target. If this happens consistently, it may be a sign that your calorie target is too high and needs adjusting.

If the opposite happens and you meet your calorie target but are short on protein, do not eat extra calories to get more protein.

Beyond the minimum amounts of dietary fat and carbohydrate you need for optimal health and performance, how much you consume of each is mostly a matter of personal preference.

Because of this, some people prefer to only track their calorie and protein intake. While this can work, we recommend setting specific fat and carbohydrate targets to help with planning, but not overly worrying if some days you eat more carbohydrate and less fat, or vice-versa.

▶ Aim to meet your fat and carbohydrate targets, but do not worry if you miss them, provided you still meet your protein and calorie goals.

THE HUMAN BODY IS REMARKABLY RESILIENT, AND YOU WILL NOT LOSE MUSCLE OR DEVELOP A NUTRIENT DEFICIENCY IF YOU DEVIATE FROM YOUR TARGETS FOR ONE DAY (BUT CONSISTENTLY MISSING YOUR TARGETS CAN CAUSE PROBLEMS).

Q2 : DOES 100G OF CHICKEN EQUAL 100G OF PROTEIN?

QUICK ANSWER:
No. There is a difference between the gross (total) weight of a food and the amount of protein, fat and carbohydrate it contains per serving.

Why?

Although many people think of foods as being 100% 'protein', 'fat' or 'carbohydrate', there are very few single macronutrient foods.

Apart from certain confectionary items (which are pure carbohydrate) and oils (which are pure fat), most foods consist of at least two macronutrients. For example, fatty protein sources like salmon contain both protein and fat.

Almost all foods contain at least some water too, which also adds to the gross (total) weight.

As a result, calculating serving sizes to meet a macronutrient target is not as straightforward as weighing a food you think of as being a good source of a specific macronutrient.

For example:

▶ 150g of chicken is not 150g of protein.

▶ 20g of almonds is not 20g of fat.

▶ 200g of rice is not 200g of carbohydrate.

You can find out the protein, fat or carbohydrate content of a food by looking at the nutrition label (typically listed as the amount per 100g) or by searching MFP.

Once you have this information, you can work out the serving sizes you need to meet your macronutrient targets – do not worry, this is easy to do on MFP.

Q3 : WHAT IF A FOOD DOES NOT HAVE A NUTRITION LABEL?

QUICK ANSWER:
Search MFP or online for a similar product from a trusted supplier, e.g. supermarket, and use this nutritional information instead.

Why?

Not all foods will have nutrition labels. For example, if you buy meat from the butchers or vegetables from a market stall.

In such cases, you can use the nutrition values for a similar product provided by a different (but trusted) supplier. For example, if you buy a sirloin steak from your local butcher, you can use the nutrition values for a packaged sirloin steak sold at a supermarket.

You can find this information by searching MFP and most supermarkets now have online stores you can search.

Q4 : SHOULD I WEIGH MY FOOD BEFORE OR AFTER COOKING?

QUICK ANSWER:
Weigh foods before cooking and calculate serving sizes based on uncooked nutrition values.

Why?

When reading nutrition labels, you will notice that they specify if the values provided apply to the food in a cooked or uncooked state.

This is an important distinction, as changes in the fluid content of foods during the cooking process can have a big impact on the calorie and macronutrient content of a serving.

When cooking meat and fish, fluids leak out meaning they are lighter after cooking. In contrast, starchy carbohydrates like rice and pasta absorb water during the cooking process.

The table below shows how 100g of uncooked chicken breast contains fewer calories and less protein than an equivalent serving of cooked chicken breast, whereas the reverse is true for the calorie and carbohydrate content of cooked and uncooked basmati rice.

The difference between the calorie and macronutrient totals for cooked versus uncooked chicken (and lean protein sources in general) are relatively minor. However, confusing the cooked and uncooked values for starchy carbohydrates and fatty protein sources can have a much bigger impact on your total calorie intake.

When selecting between the cooked and uncooked method it is important to consider:

▶ Nearly all nutrition labels now use the uncooked method.

▶ How long you cook foods for will vary slightly each time and affect the cooked weight.

▶ Weighing individual components of mixed meals, e.g. stir fries, after cooking can get very messy!

▶ It is a lot easier for certain cooked foods to get 'lost' on the way to the food scale and end up in your mouth.

As a result, we recommend weighing foods prior to cooking and calculating serving sizes based on the uncooked nutrition values.

WHEN COOKING MEAT AND FISH, FLUIDS LEAK OUT MEANING THEY ARE LIGHTER AFTER COOKING. IN CONTRAST, STARCHY CARBOHYDRATES LIKE RICE AND PASTA ABSORB WATER DURING THE COOKING PROCESS.

FOOD	100G CHICKEN BREAST		100G BASMATI RICE	
	PROTEIN	CALORIES	CARBOHYDRATE	CALORIES
Cooked	28g	145kcal	25g	120kcal
Uncooked	23g	120kcal	75g	350kcal

Q5 : DO I NEED TO WEIGH ALL MY FOOD?

QUICK ANSWER:
No. You can use the weight listed on the packaging for meat, fruit and vegetables. But, always weigh portions of fat sources when extracting servings from a bulk package, e.g. tub or bottle.

Why?

You do not need to weigh foods if the weight is listed on the packaging.

Sometimes, you will know the weight of a food but only plan on eating part of it now and saving the rest for later. In such cases, make a note of the total weight, cook the food, and then 'eyeball' your serving size.

For example, if you decide to batch cook 400g of chicken breast for two meals, cook all the chicken and then roughly split it into two servings after cooking.

This approach works well when batch-cooking fresh foods like meat, fruit and vegetables that you will eat relatively close together, for example, later in the same day or week. You may end up eating slightly more at one meal and less at another, but you will balance out any measurement error by the end of the day or week.

In contrast, we recommend taking a more measured approach when extracting servings of more calorie-dense foods like nuts, rice and pasta. Not many people have the self-control or precision to dip their hand into a bag of nuts and pull out the exact serving size required.

These foods also have longer shelf lives and often come in bulk-packages. Although any measurement error will eventually balance out, this may take several weeks, or even months, and cause you to overeat in the short-term.

Q6 : HOW CAN I CALCULATE SERVING SIZES MYSELF?

QUICK ANSWER:
There is a simple calculation you can use to work out serving sizes, but we recommend letting MFP do the maths for you!

Why?

You can manually calculate the amount of food you need to meet a specific macronutrient target using the following formula:

$$\frac{\text{MACRONUTRIENT TARGET}}{\div \text{ AMOUNT PER 100G } (\textit{in decimal form})}$$

To convert the macronutrient content per 100g into decimal form, you need to divide it by 100. For example, 25g of protein would be 0.25.

So, if you wanted to calculate how much chicken you needed to eat for 40g of protein:

1. Check the nutrition label to see how much protein chicken has per 100g of uncooked weight, e.g. 25g protein per 100g of uncooked weight.

2. Complete the following calculation:
   40 / 0.25 = 160g of uncooked chicken breast.

In reality, you will very rarely need to manually calculate serving sizes, as MFP does the maths for you!

QUICK ANSWER:
No. Always use grams as the unit of measurement when weighing foods and recording them in MFP.

Why?

Most nutrition labels list serving sizes in terms of a standardised unit of volume, e.g. cup or tablespoon, followed by the weight in grams.

We recommend weighing your food where possible, as the volume-based method of measuring serving sizes can be very inconsistent.

One cup, tablespoon, scoop or any other measurement of volume can produce very different serving sizes (in terms of weight and therefore calorie content) depending on:

▶ The form of food, e.g. whole, chopped or mashed vegetables.

▶ How you pack the food into the measuring device.

▶ Individual variances in the size of measuring devices.

The volume-based method is also prone to abuse with certain hyper-palatable foods and can lead to hidden calories sneaking into your diet.

For example, the image below shows how two tablespoons of almond nut butter can have vastly different calorie contents.

When recording items in MFP, always select an entry that allows you to use grams as the unit of measurement (some entries are based on food volume, e.g. cups).

Certain entries will not have an option for grams. In such cases, select another option from the search results.

THE VOLUME-BASED METHOD IS ALSO PRONE TO ABUSE WITH CERTAIN HYPER-PALATABLE FOODS AND CAN LEAD TO HIDDEN CALORIES SNEAKING INTO YOUR DIET.

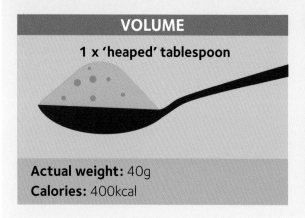

VOLUME

1 x 'heaped' tablespoon

Actual weight: 40g
Calories: 400kcal

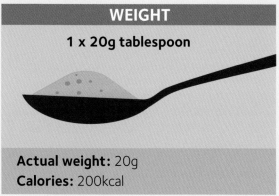

WEIGHT

1 x 20g tablespoon

Actual weight: 20g
Calories: 200kcal

HOW TO WRITE A MEAL PLAN

THE AIM OF THIS SECTION IS TO SHOW YOU HOW TO WRITE A MEAL PLAN THAT FITS WITH YOUR SCHEDULE, MEETS YOUR DAILY NUTRITION TARGETS AND PROPERLY FUELS YOUR WORKOUTS.

We have broken down the daily meal planning process into six key steps and will guide you through each one in detail.

To follow along step-by-step, you will need access to MFP and the transformation food tables.

STEP 1:
SCHEDULE YOUR MEALS

The first step in scheduling your meals is to decide how many times you will eat each day.

A key point to make here is that the total amount of food consumed within a 24-hour window is far more important than your meal frequency or the specific timing of your meals.

From experience, we find that three to five meals work best. Where you fall on this range will depend on your own personal preferences and what fits with your schedule.

If you are new to meal planning, we recommend starting with four meals spaced evenly throughout your day in three to five hour intervals.

For most people, a four-meal schedule will mean an early morning breakfast, lunch, dinner and either a mid-morning or mid-afternoon meal.

Try to schedule regular times for your meals. Eating at roughly the same times will make following the diet part of your routine and help with hunger and cravings, as you will know when your next meal is coming.

Scheduling your meals is important, but do not worry if:

▶ Your schedule does not allow for evenly spaced meals throughout your day.

▶ Something crops up and you have to move meals forwards or backwards from their planned times.

The most important thing is to create a meal plan that meets your daily nutrition targets and that you can follow consistently. For long-term success, your meal schedule must fit with your lifestyle, not the other way around!

> **FROM EXPERIENCE, WE FIND THAT THREE TO FIVE MEALS WORK BEST. WHERE YOU FALL ON THIS RANGE WILL DEPEND ON YOUR OWN PERSONAL PREFERENCES AND WHAT FITS WITH YOUR SCHEDULE.**

ACTION

Select your meal frequency/times and add them to your diary.

STEP 2:
PLAN YOUR PROTEIN

Meeting your daily protein target should be your main priority, but research also suggests that spreading your intake over multiple protein feedings is best for muscle growth.

To optimise your protein intake:

▶ Include a protein source with each of your meals.

▶ Aim for a 20-50g serving of protein per meal.

▶ Aim to get most of your daily protein intake from animal-origin sources as they contain all the EAAs your body needs for optimal health and building muscle.

▶ Consider limiting fatty protein sources to one serving (20-50g) per day, so you can include a greater volume of food in your diet.

▶ Consider limiting protein supplements to one serving (20-50g) per day and use whole food sources to meet the rest of your target.

You can make adjustments to serving sizes within the 20-50g range. For example, you may prefer a smaller serving in the morning if you struggle for appetite, e.g. 20g, and a larger serving in the evening, e.g. 50g.

Some protein sources also tend to be more convenient and palatable at certain times of the day than others. For example, most people have time to prepare eggs for breakfast, but may not find the prospect of white fish very appealing.

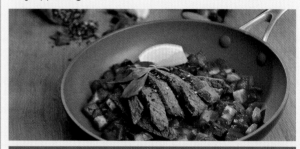

ACTION

Allocate your protein target and select a protein source for each meal.

STEP 3:
PLAN YOUR FATS

The next step is to allocate the remainder of your fat target. Remember, you will already have used a portion of this meeting your protein target.

There are no specific timing requirements for dietary fats, therefore you can add them to your meal plan based on personal preference.

THERE ARE NO SPECIFIC TIMING REQUIREMENTS FOR DIETARY FATS, THEREFORE YOU CAN ADD THEM TO YOUR MEAL PLAN BASED ON PERSONAL PREFERENCE.

A good starting point is to spread your intake evenly across each meal to help add texture and flavour.

To optimise your fat intake:

▶ Include a balance of all three types of fats (SFAs, MUFAs, PUFAs) in your diet. You can do this by using a varied selection of the sources listed in the fat table to meet your target.

▶ Aim to use fatty fish as your fatty protein source two to three times per week or take a daily fish oil supplement.

ACTION

Add fat sources to your meal plan to meet your fat target.

STEP 4:
PLAN YOUR CARBOHYDRATES

When allocating your carbohydrate target you should prioritise including non-starchy vegetables in your meal plan, followed by fruit and then starchy vegetables/grains.

We recommend including vegetables with every meal, but there are no specific timing requirements for fruit or starchy vegetables/grains.

Fruits make a great low-calorie snack option, or you can include them as part of a meal.

Regarding starchy vegetables/grains, some of our clients prefer to save them for the evening when they have more time to prepare and enjoy them.

Alternatively, you can spread them evenly throughout your day and we have provided example carbohydrate-based breakfast, lunch and dinner options in the transformation recipes.

To optimise your carbohydrate intake:

▶ Aim to fill half your plate with non-starchy vegetables at every meal. This equates to roughly 100-200g of uncooked weight per meal.

▶ Add one to two servings (roughly 100kcal per serving) of fruit per day to your meal plan as a snack or part of a meal.

▶ Once you have added non-starchy vegetables and fruit, add starchy vegetables/grains to your meal plan to meet your carbohydrate target.

▶ You do not need to track your fibre intake if you include a variety of vegetables, fruits and whole grains in your meal plan.

REGARDING STARCHY VEGETABLES/ GRAINS, SOME OF OUR CLIENTS PREFER TO SAVE THEM FOR THE EVENING WHEN THEY HAVE MORE TIME TO PREPARE AND ENJOY THEM.

ACTION
Add carbohydrate sources to your meal plan to meet your carbohydrate target.

STEP 5:
ADD DRINKS AND CONDIMENTS TO YOUR MEAL PLAN

After you have allocated your macronutrients, the next step is to add drinks and condiments to your meal plan.

To optimise your fluid intake:

▶ Aim for at least two litres of fluids per day and follow the hydration habits outlined in the 'Transformation Foods' section.

▶ Use the minimum effective caffeine dose and avoid it from the early afternoon (2-3pm) onwards.

▶ You do not have to include diet sodas in your meal plan but should not feel guilty about doing so in moderation either.

▶ Limit alcohol intake to 10-15% of your daily calorie target one to two times per week.

Herbs, seasonings and spices are all great ways to add flavour to your meals. Check out the transformation recipes for ideas on how to include them in your meal plan.

ACTION
Add drinks and condiments to your meal plan.

STEP 6:
MAKE FINAL ADJUSTMENTS

Once you have scheduled and planned your meals, the final step is to make sure the calorie and macronutrient totals for each meal add up to meet your daily targets.

You may have to adjust certain serving sizes up or down slightly, but remember that the macronutrient ratios do not have to be perfect.

When making your final adjustments:

▶ Aim to meet your calorie target within a +/- 50kcal range.

▶ Aim to meet your protein target within a +/- 10g range.

▶ Aim to meet your fat and carbohydrate targets, but do not worry if you miss them, provided you still meet your protein and calorie goals.

ACTION

Double check your macronutrient/calorie totals and make any final adjustments to serving sizes.

WORKOUT NUTRITION

There are three potential eating windows around a workout: pre, intra (during) and post-workout. Here is a summary of the key points you need to consider when writing your meal plan:

PRE-WORKOUT

If training during the daytime, we recommend timing your workout to fall between two of your normal meals.

Aim to leave at least one hour between the pre-workout meal and the start of your workout to avoid stomach upset.

INTRA-WORKOUT

If proper pre-workout nutrition is in place and you are training for 60 minutes or less, then you do not need to consume any additional protein, fat or carbohydrate during your workout. Instead, your primary concern should be remaining properly hydrated.

POST-WORKOUT

For years, it was widely believed that you must consume some form of post-workout nutrition as close as possible to the end of your workout.

However, we now know that the need for immediate post-workout nutrition is less critical, because:

▶ It takes several hours to digest a meal, therefore the nutrients from your pre-workout meal will be available to support the post-workout recovery process.

▶ Research has now proven that resistance training to failure causes an increased anabolic (growth) response to protein consumption that lasts for up to 24-hours.

▶ You only need to rapidly replenish your body's carbohydrate stores if you are training the same muscle groups to exhaustion twice in one day. In most cases, you will have at least 24 hours before you re-train a specific muscle group.

This does not mean that you should completely disregard post-workout nutrition. There is no benefit to delaying the recovery process and many of our clients enjoy a well-earned protein shake after a challenging workout.

If you are training first thing in the morning, or at some other point during the day where you have not eaten for more than four to six hours, we recommend having a small (roughly 200kcal), easy-to-digest and protein-based pre-workout snack. For example, a protein shake and piece of fruit.

Alternatively, if you prefer to train fasted and it does not affect your performance, make sure to eat soon after your workout finishes.

ANDREW

DAILY TARGETS

Protein: 180g **Fat:** 70g
Carbohydrate: 285g **Calories:** 2,490kcal

MEAL 1 | TIME: 7 AM

Protein: 55g **Fat:** 31g **Carbs:** 58g **Calories:** 754kcal

FOOD GROUP	FOOD	UNCOOKED SERVING (g)
Protein Source	Sirloin Steak	145g
Fat Source	Almonds	15g
Non-Starchy Veg	Mixed Veg	150g
Fruit	–	–
Starchy Veg/Grains	Oatmeal	80g
Drinks	Black Coffee and Water	–

MEAL 2 | TIME: 12 NOON

Protein: 45g **Fat:** 9g **Carbs:** 60g **Calories:** 507kcal

FOOD GROUP	FOOD	UNCOOKED SERVING (g)
Protein Source	Chicken Breast	150g
Fat Source	Feta Cheese	20g
Non-Starchy Veg	Mixed Salad	150g
Fruit	Banana	–
Starchy Veg/Grains	Brown Rice	70g
Drinks	Water and Green Tea	–

MEAL 3 | TIME: 4 PM

Protein: 51g **Fat:** 10g **Carbs:** 69g **Calories:** 586kcal

FOOD GROUP	FOOD	UNCOOKED SERVING (g)
Protein Source	Chicken Breast	150g
Fat Source	Feta Cheese	20g
Non-Starchy Veg	Mixed Salad	150g
Fruit	Banana	100g
Starchy Veg/Grains	Brown Rice	70g
Drinks	Water	–

MEAL 4 | TIME: 8 PM

Protein: 37g **Fat:** 18g **Carbs:** 78g **Calories:** 634kcal

FOOD GROUP	FOOD	UNCOOKED SERVING (g)
Protein Source	Cod Fillet	180g
Fat Source	Olive Oil	15ml
Non-Starchy Veg	Mixed Veg	150g
Fruit	Blueberries	100g
Starchy Veg/Grains	Sweet Potato	300g
Drinks	Water	–

DAILY TOTALS

Protein: 188g **Fat:** 68g **Carbs:** 265g **Calories:** 2,481kcal

NOTES

Four evenly spaced meals from 7am to 8pm.

Each meal includes an animal-origin protein source and contains between 20-50g of protein.

Andrew had to adjust his protein source serving sizes when he realised that fat sources, e.g. feta cheese, and carbohydrate sources, e.g. oatmeal, also contain protein.

Andrew did not include a protein shake in his meal plan as he prefers to eat, rather than drink, his protein.

Meal 2 and 3 are the same because Andrew makes one big chicken salad every night and splits it into two portions.

Protein sources used up 10g (14%) of Andrew's fat target, leaving 60g to allocate to fat sources.

Andrew spread his fat intake evenly across the day and used a variety of sources, e.g. adding feta cheese to his salad and olive oil to his cod fillet.

Every meal includes a serving of non-starchy vegetables.

Andrew included a serving of fruit with meal 3 and 4, so he could have something sweet after his main meal.

Non-starchy vegetables and fruit used up 50g (18%) of Andrew's carbohydrate target, leaving 215g to allocate to starchy vegetables/grains.

Andrew's carbohydrate target is relatively high, so he spread it evenly across all four meals to avoid huge serving sizes.

Andrew did not hit any of his macronutrient targets to the gram but was within +/- 50kcal of his calorie target and +/-10g of his protein target.

On training days, Andrew moves meal 2 and 3 forwards slightly and trains between meal 3 and 4.

JENNY

DAILY TARGETS

Protein: 105g **Fat:** 65g
Carbohydrate: 160g **Calories:** 1,640kcal

MEAL 1 | TIME: 7 AM

Protein: 20g **Fat:** 13g **Carbs:** 23g **Calories:** 285kcal

FOOD GROUP	FOOD	UNCOOKED SERVING (g)
Protein Source	0% Fat Greek Yoghurt	150g
Fat Source	Walnuts	20g
Non-Starchy Veg	–	–
Fruit	Blueberries	100g
Starchy Veg/Grains	–	–
Drinks	Black Coffee and Water	–

MEAL 2 | TIME: 11 AM

Protein: 32g **Fat:** 24g **Carbs:** 52g **Calories:** 566kcal

FOOD GROUP	FOOD	UNCOOKED SERVING (g)
Protein Source	Turkey Breast	100g
Fat Source	Avocado	100g
Non-Starchy Veg	Mixed Veg	150g
Fruit	–	–
Starchy Veg/Grains	Sweet Potato	200g
Drinks	Water and Fruit Tea	–

MEAL 3 | TIME: 3 PM

Protein: 29g **Fat:** 10g **Carbs:** 16g **Calories:** 283kcal

FOOD GROUP	FOOD	UNCOOKED SERVING (g)
Protein Source	Whey Protein Shake	25g
Fat Source	85% Dark Chocolate	15g
Non-Starchy Veg	–	–
Fruit	Banana	100g
Starchy Veg/Grains	–	–
Drinks	Water	–

MEAL 4 | TIME: 7 PM

Protein: 34g **Fat:** 14g **Carbs:** 52g **Calories:** 472kcal

FOOD GROUP	FOOD	UNCOOKED SERVING (g)
Protein Source	Sirloin Steak	100g
Fat Source	–	–
Non-Starchy Veg	Mixed Veg	150g
Fruit	–	–
Starchy Veg/Grains	Brown Rice	60g
Drinks	Water	–

DAILY TOTALS

Protein: 115g **Fat:** 61g **Carbs:** 143g **Calories:** 1,590kcal

NOTES

Four evenly spaced meals from 7am to 7pm.

Each meal includes an animal-origin protein source and contains between 20-50g of protein.

Jenny struggles for appetite early in the morning and finds Greek yoghurt more palatable than meat or fish.

Jenny only included one fatty protein source, sirloin steak, so that she could spread her fat target over a greater volume of foods, e.g. walnuts and avocado.

Jenny included a protein shake in her meal plan as it is an easy-to-prepare meal while at work.

Protein sources used up 13g (20%) of Jenny's fat target, leaving 52g to allocate to fat sources.

Jenny spread her fat intake evenly across the day and used a variety of sources, e.g. adding walnuts to her Greek yoghurt and avocado to meal 2.

Jenny does not like the taste of fish and prefers to take a fish oil supplement.

Jenny included a serving of vegetables with meal 2 and 4 and included two servings of fruit in her meal plan.

Non-starchy vegetables and fruit used up 39g (24%) of Jenny's carbohydrate target, leaving 121g to allocate to starchy vegetables/grains.

Jenny's carbohydrate target is lower than Andrew's, and she chose to allocate most of it to her two main meals (meal 2 and 4).

Jenny did not hit any of her macronutrient targets to the gram but was within +/- 50kcal of her calorie target and +/-10g of her protein target.

On training days, Jenny has a mid-morning snack and pushes meal 2, 3 and 4 back slightly so she can train during her lunch break.

ADAPTING THE MEAL PLAN: DINING OUT

—

SO FAR, WE HAVE FOCUSED ON HOW TO CREATE A MEAL PLAN FOR DAYS WHEN YOU ARE PREPARING ALL YOUR OWN MEALS.

However, there will be times during your transformation when you do not have complete control over what you get to eat. For example, you may have a work lunch with colleagues or dinner out with friends.

This section will explain how you can adapt your meal plan to factor in dining out, while continuing to make progress towards your transformation.

STEP 1:
PLAN AHEAD

The biggest mistake people make when dining out is not planning far enough in advance.

To avoid this, ask yourself the following question at the end of each week:

"How many work or social events do I have scheduled for next week that may affect my progress?"

Identifying any events in advance will give you plenty of time to formulate a plan and adapt the rest of your week if necessary.

When reviewing your upcoming week, you should consider:

Sometimes Eating at Home Works Best

Although food will be available at certain events, there may not be an expectation for you to eat. For example, many of our clients regularly attend evening drinks parties where there is typically a buffet or canapes on offer.

In such cases, we recommend eating at home before the event. Make sure to time your meal close to the event as this will help you to stay strong in the face of temptation.

You Can Socialise Without Dining Out

For many people, dining out is the default option for networking with colleagues or socialising with friends and family.

While we certainly do not want to discourage this, you should also consider non-food related activities like coffee meetings, bowling or the cinema.

Tell People About Your Transformation

Some people reading this will be in the fortunate position where their friend, partner or relative prepares a large proportion of their food for them.

If this is the case, you need to have a conversation with them before starting your transformation so they can prepare meals that fit with your goals.

Even if you prepare your own meals, we recommend updating people that you regularly socialise and interact with on your transformation plans so they can support you along the way.

STEP 2:
CHOOSE THE RESTAURANT AND GET THE MENU

Once you have identified how many times you will be dining out during the upcoming week, the next step is to review where you will be eating.

If possible, try to take the lead and suggest a venue that you know offers healthy options.

This should be relatively straightforward to research as most restaurants share sample menus on their website or will be happy to send a copy if you get in touch.

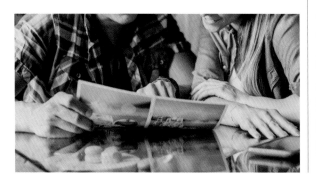

A top tip here is to find go-to options for different dining out occasions that fit with your meal plan.

Do a little research and identify a go-to medium-priced restaurant for casual meals with friends, a higher-priced restaurant for special occasions and a fast-food chain, café or supermarket for convenience.

Even if you cannot influence the choice of restaurant, you should still make an effort to get a copy of the menu in advance. This is important as it gives you time to properly review the menu and make a decision without any peer pressure from fellow diners.

THIS SHOULD BE RELATIVELY STRAIGHTFORWARD TO RESEARCH AS MOST RESTAURANTS SHARE SAMPLE MENUS ON THEIR WEBSITE OR WILL BE HAPPY TO SEND A COPY IF YOU GET IN TOUCH.

STEP 3:
SELECT YOUR MEAL

So, what do you do once you have the menu?

Identify the Protein Sources
The number one rule to follow when dining out during a transformation is to make sure that protein is the main component of the meal.

For example, a steak dinner is a protein-rich meal, whereas protein is just a topping on a pizza.

When deciding between protein sources, we recommend choosing the leanest option. For example, go for a fillet steak, rather than a sirloin or rib-eye.

An unavoidable truth of dining out is that any meal you order will almost always contain more calories than the same meal prepared at home.

You may care about controlling your calories, but the chef's priority is making food taste good, which often means using plenty of calorie-dense, flavour-adding ingredients like oil, butter and cream.

We call these 'hidden calories', and while they are difficult to spot, they can have a big impact on the calorie total of a meal.

Selecting a lean protein source helps to control the total calorie count, as any hidden calories are added on top of a lean protein source, rather than a higher-calorie fatty protein source.

Skip Dessert and Go with Starter/Main or Main Only

Almost all restaurants have the option to choose a starter, main course and dessert.

Depending on how many calories you have allocated for the meal, we recommend ordering either a main course only, or a starter and a main.

Restaurant dessert options are almost always calorie bombs. In contrast, most starters typically come in small serving sizes and there is normally a protein-based option available.

In fact, if a starter looks like a good option, you could order it as your main and fill out the meal with side dishes.

And what should you do if everybody else orders a dessert? Have a coffee (decaffeinated if eating late) or tea, and enjoy the conversation!

Modify the Menu

If you see an option that is close to being a good choice, ask the server if they can modify it. Common examples include asking to replace fries with salad and for dressings and sauces to be served on the side.

Another modification you can make is to order a side of vegetables to bulk out your meal. However, vegetables are not automatically low-calorie options when dining out, especially if fried or served in butter or creamy sauces.

The menu description will not always mention this, so check with the server and ask for them to be steamed or served 'dry'. Alternatively, the safest bet is to order a salad with the dressing on the side, as this involves no cooking.

The final modification is to remember that you do not have to clear your plate. Some restaurants are very generous with serving sizes (especially with carbohydrate sources like rice and potatoes), or only offer large serving sizes, such as massive steaks.

In such cases, do not be afraid to only eat a normal sized portion and either leave the rest, share with a fellow diner or ask to take the leftovers home.

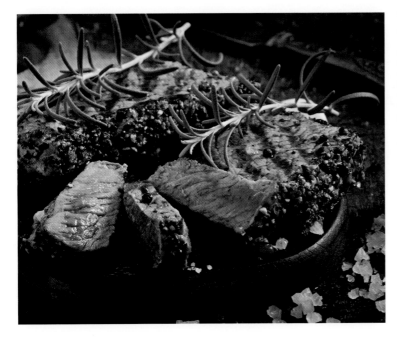

THE NUMBER ONE RULE TO FOLLOW WHEN DINING OUT DURING A TRANSFORMATION IS TO MAKE SURE THAT PROTEIN IS THE MAIN COMPONENT OF THE MEAL.

FOR EXAMPLE, A STEAK DINNER IS A PROTEIN-RICH MEAL, WHEREAS PROTEIN IS JUST A TOPPING ON A PIZZA.

STEP 4:
ADAPT YOUR MEAL PLAN

On days when you are not dining out, the meal planning process starts by scheduling your meals and selecting your protein sources.

On days when you are dining out, you should start by selecting your order (step 3), and then estimating how much of your daily food intake this takes up. You can then plan how to spread the remainder of your calories over the rest of your day.

The first place to check when estimating the calorie content of a meal is online, as a lot of restaurants now list nutritional information on their website.

If the information is not available, try looking for a similar meal on the menu of a restaurant that does share this information.

Failing this, you will have to 'guesstimate' the calorie content of the meal, by researching the individual ingredients.

This is much easier to do when you choose simple menu options, like steak and vegetables, compared to complex, multi-ingredient meals like a curry or lasagne. Your estimate will also be more accurate, as restaurants typically list the serving sizes for protein sources on the menu.

You then need to adjust your estimate to account for any hidden calories. From experience, the easiest way to do this is to add 25% to your calorie estimate for the meal. For example, 400kcal becomes 500kcal, 500kcal becomes 625kcal, and so on.

The next step is to plan the rest of your day by following the steps outlined below:

1. Subtract your calorie guestimate from your daily calorie target to calculate your revised calorie target.

2. Subtract your protein guestimate from your daily protein target to calculate your revised protein target.

3. Follow the meal planning steps for non-dining out days to plan the rest of your day.

Note: you can assume that the +25% adjustment came purely from fat and adjust your fat target accordingly, or just focus on hitting your protein and calorie target for the day.

If the meal is bigger than expected, simply adapt your serving sizes later in the day and you will know for next time.

STEP 5:
ENJOY THE MEAL

The final step in adapting your meal plan for dining out is to remember to enjoy the meal!

Feeling included and spending time with your friends and family is incredibly important when dieting and avoiding social occasions for fear of falling off the wagon is an unnecessary worry.

Ultimately, your rate of progress will determine if your approach to dining out is effective or if you need to make a change.

FEELING INCLUDED AND SPENDING TIME WITH YOUR FRIENDS AND FAMILY IS INCREDIBLY IMPORTANT WHEN DIETING AND AVOIDING SOCIAL OCCASIONS FOR FEAR OF FALLING OFF THE WAGON IS AN UNNECESSARY WORRY.

ADAPTING THE MEAL PLAN: REFEEDS

THE NEXT MODIFICATION YOU CAN MAKE TO YOUR MEAL PLAN IS TO INCLUDE A REFEED.

This section will outline exactly what a refeed is, the benefits and how to include them in your meal plan.

What is a Refeed?

A refeed is a planned period of increased calorie intake while dieting that can last anywhere from a few hours up to a few days. The focus of this section will be on single-day (24-hour) refeeds.

Why Refeed?

Refeeds and Metabolic Adaptation

The general idea behind a refeed is that it is not always good for your body to be in a calorie deficit and it can benefit from a break.

Whenever you restrict your calorie intake for an extended period and lose a significant amount of body fat, you will most likely experience the effects of several adaptations made by your body to try and prevent further fat loss and conserve energy.

Remember, your body cannot tell the difference between a voluntary diet and genuine food scarcity.

These adaptations (collectively known as 'metabolic adaptation') can be both psychological and physiological and include:

▶ Reduced energy expenditure from NEAT (you move around less).

▶ Changes in hormone levels that promote increased hunger, decreased metabolic rate and increased risk of LBM loss.

▶ Increased cravings and food-focused behaviour.

In theory, a refeed signals to your body that energy is now available, there is no need to worry, and that fat loss can continue uninterrupted.

It is unlikely that a single-day refeed can completely reverse adaptations that take several weeks of caloric restriction to develop. However, including them at regular intervals may help slow down the rate at which they occur.

Refeeds and Performance

Your body has a limited capacity for storing glycogen which is your muscle's primary fuel source during high-intensity exercise.

Resistance training and caloric restriction both deplete your body's glycogen stores, which can negatively impact your workout performance over time.

Including a refeed the day before a tough workout will replenish your glycogen stores and provide the energy you need to power through.

Refeeds and Psychological Breaks

Arguably the most important benefit of a refeed is that it provides a mental break from dieting, specifically:

▶ Scheduling refeeds in advance can break up long periods of dieting into more manageable blocks and give you something to look forward to.

▶ Refeeds can add variety to your diet and allow you to include foods that you may have temporarily restricted, but sorely miss!

▶ No diet will ever be completely distraction-free, and you can time refeeds to coincide with events like birthday meals and nights out with friends.

In summary, single-day refeeds cannot magically increase your rate of fat loss or completely counteract metabolic adaptations that occur when dieting for extended periods.

However, they do provide a short-term boost in workout performance as well as several psychological benefits that make them worthy of consideration.

Refeed Frequency
– Do You Really Need a Refeed?

A key point to make about all the adaptations to dieting discussed so far is that the extent to which they occur depends on several factors, including:

1. How long you have been dieting.

2. Your starting body fat percentage.

3. The size of calorie deficit.

If you are just starting your diet, have relatively high body fat levels (no sign of visible abs yet) and are taking a sensible approach, then you do not really need a refeed.

Including refeeds becomes more important when you have been dieting for several weeks, have lost a lot of body fat and are struggling with the effects of what experienced dieters call 'diet fatigue'.

It is also important to consider that not everybody responds favourably to refeeds.

If you are starting a training and nutrition program after years of poor eating habits, then taking breaks early in the process can disrupt the creation of new healthy eating habits.

And although this should not be an issue if you follow the advice outlined in this guide, some dieters become overly fixated on the refeed day, which increases the chances of them overeating.

IF YOU ARE STARTING A TRAINING AND NUTRITION PROGRAM AFTER YEARS OF POOR EATING HABITS, THEN TAKING BREAKS EARLY IN THE PROCESS CAN DISRUPT THE CREATION OF NEW HEALTHY EATING HABITS.

Refeed Recommendations

The only real way to know how you respond to a refeed is to test it out. To do this, we recommend:

▶ Start by establishing basic healthy eating habits and do not include a refeed for the first three weeks of your transformation.

▶ Schedule your first refeed for a day of your choice in week 4.

▶ If you enjoy the refeed and find that it helps restore some physical and mental energy, continue to schedule one refeed day every 7-14 days.

▶ If you find that It disrupts your routine and makes it difficult to get back on track, you do not need to include a refeed.

Most clients tend to enjoy refeeds, and at the very least you should view it as a nutritional insurance policy to help navigate cravings, social events or times when you have limited food choices.

How to Refeed

When to Refeed

There is no specific day you must perform a refeed on and it can change each time.

Here are some starting suggestions:

▶ Schedule the refeed for the day before your toughest workout of the week.

▶ If performing a refeed to help navigate a social situation, then time it to coincide.

▶ Some clients prefer to schedule refeeds for a day they are not working so they have more time to prepare and enjoy the extra calories.

Refeed Size

▶ The aim is to increase your calories to a point where you are no longer in a calorie deficit.

▶ To keep things simple, we recommend setting the refeed calorie target as the maintenance calorie value you estimated earlier.

▶ Having a target to aim for is essential, rather than adopting a 'cheat day' mentality and eating whatever takes your fancy. Increasing your calories to maintenance is like pressing the pause button on fat loss, whereas a cheat day can easily erase several days of dieting!

What to Eat

▶ We recommend aiming for your normal protein target (but you can eat more), and the remaining calories can come from any food or non-alcoholic drink of your choice.

▶ A common mistake people make is trying to fit as much 'junk food' into the refeed day as possible. The problems here are that they often end up exceeding the refeed target and struggle to return to their 'normal diet' the following day.

▶ For the best results, we recommend including some treats, but mainly eating more of the same foods that you have built the rest of your meal plan around.

HOW TO CALCULATE YOUR REFEED TARGETS

STEP 1:
SET REFEED CALORIE TARGET

Set the refeed calorie target as the maintenance calorie value you estimated earlier.

STEP 2:
SET MACRONUTRIENT TARGETS

Aim for your normal protein target (but you can eat more), and the remaining calories can come from a macronutrient distribution of your choice.

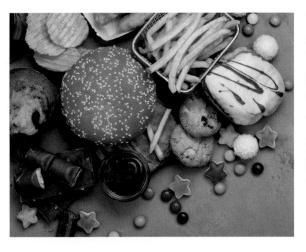

A COMMON MISTAKE PEOPLE MAKE IS TRYING TO FIT AS MUCH 'JUNK FOOD' INTO THE REFEED DAY AS POSSIBLE. THE PROBLEMS HERE ARE THAT THEY OFTEN END UP EXCEEDING THE REFEED TARGET AND STRUGGLE TO RETURN TO THEIR 'NORMAL DIET' THE FOLLOWING DAY.

ADAPTING THE MEAL PLAN: CALORIE SHIFTING

THE FINAL MODIFICATION YOU CAN MAKE TO YOUR MEAL PLAN IS TO SHIFT CALORIES BETWEEN DAYS WHILE MAINTAINING YOUR TARGET WEEKLY CALORIE AVERAGE.

This section will explain how you can make small adjustments to your daily calorie target to stay on track during your transformation.

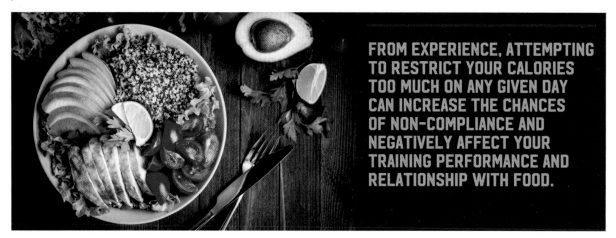

FROM EXPERIENCE, ATTEMPTING TO RESTRICT YOUR CALORIES TOO MUCH ON ANY GIVEN DAY CAN INCREASE THE CHANCES OF NON-COMPLIANCE AND NEGATIVELY AFFECT YOUR TRAINING PERFORMANCE AND RELATIONSHIP WITH FOOD.

Although it is important to aim for your daily nutrition targets, it is your average intake over a longer period that will determine your progress.

This explains why you can include a higher calorie refeed day in your program and still make progress. It is also why one 'bad day' cannot undo several weeks of consistent dieting.

We typically prefer to aim for the same nutrition targets each day, as this simplifies meal planning and helps make it part of your routine.

However, there can be times where shifting calories between days (while maintaining your target weekly average) can help you to stay on track, for example, having extra calories to navigate social situations.

From experience, attempting to restrict your calories too much on any given day can increase the chances of non-compliance and negatively affect your training performance and relationship with food.

As a result, we recommend:

▶ Do not reduce a single day's calorie allotment by more than 10%.

▶ Move calories from a maximum of three days per week.

▶ Move calories from rest days, rather than training days, if possible.

You can also use the above approach to correct for overeating on certain days. However, we recommend only doing this to balance out minor deviations of a couple of hundred calories.

In all other situations, chalk it up as a refeed, and refocus on meeting your normal targets.

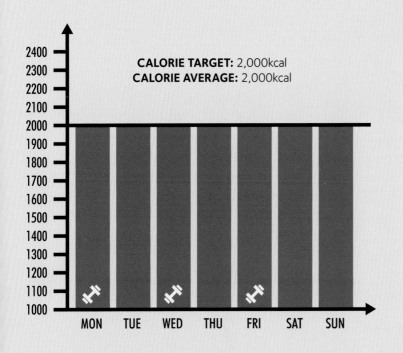

CALORIE TARGET: 2,000kcal
CALORIE AVERAGE: 2,000kcal

NORMAL WEEK

In this example, the client meets their 2,000kcal target every day and does not shift calories between days.

Calorie shifting is a useful tactic, but if you plan, you should be able to account for a lot of events like meals out within your normal target.

From week 4 onwards, you can also use refeed days (every 7–14 days) to help navigate work and social events.

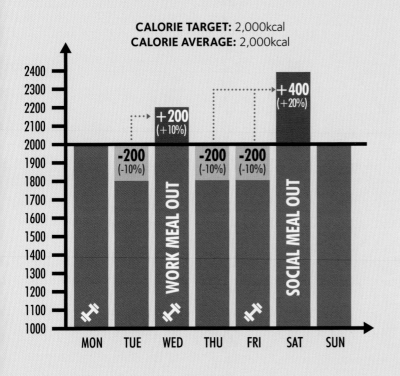

CALORIE TARGET: 2,000kcal
CALORIE AVERAGE: 2,000kcal

CALORIE SHIFTING WEEK

In this example, the client shifts calories between days but still averages 2,000kcal per day. As a result, they will achieve the same results as if they had consumed 2,000kcal every day.

The client trains on Monday, Wednesday and Friday and has managed to avoid reducing calories on all but one of these days. Limiting the reduction to 10% should stop this having a negative impact on their performance.

A common mistake to avoid is using the calorie shifting technique to free up extra calories for 'junk food' and alcohol. For best results, we recommend sticking to our guidelines for dining out.

WEEKLY MEAL PLANNING

NOW THAT YOU KNOW HOW TO CREATE AND ADAPT A DAILY MEAL PLAN, THE FINAL THING WE NEED TO COVER IS HOW TO PLAN A FULL WEEK.

We have broken down the weekly meal planning process into three key steps and will guide you through each one in detail.

For the best results, you should schedule a regular time each weekend to complete your weekly meal plan.

To follow along step-by-step, you will need to create a similar template to the one on page (p.86), or download one from our website, www.upfitness.com.

STEP 1:
PLAN YOUR WEEK

As discussed previously, at the end of each week ask yourself the following question:

"How many work or social events do I have scheduled for next week that may affect my progress?"

If you are dining out, do you have any influence over where you are dining? If you do, great, but if not, you still need to get a copy of the menu.

In addition to dining out, the weekly scan should also identify any other events, e.g. travel or late nights at work, that may disrupt your routine and need to be accounted for in your planning.

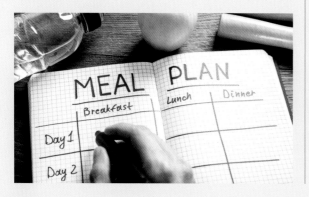

STEP 2:
SCHEDULE YOUR MEALS

The next step is to schedule your meals for the week.

Three key points to make here are:

▶ You do not have to plan your exact macronutrient and calorie intakes for each day a full week in advance. But, you should have a rough idea of the meals you will be eating.

▶ You do not have to prepare all your meals for the full week in advance. Whether you decide to batch cook, prepare food each day or use a combination of both methods is up to you – just make sure you have a plan!

▶ In the example weekly meal plan, we have kept meal frequency and timings consistent across the week. However, you may have to adapt this on days where you dine out, depending on the size and scheduled time of the meal out.

A top tip to simplify the meal planning process is to create one or two regular meals for each meal time. For example, making it part of your routine to have eggs for breakfast and a chicken salad for lunch.

This may sound boring, but you can make slight modifications to the meal each day or switch it up entirely every few weeks.

Finally, do not worry if you decide to change your plan during the week, just cross out what you did not have and make a note of what you had instead.

A TOP TIP TO SIMPLIFY THE MEAL PLANNING PROCESS IS TO CREATE ONE OR TWO REGULAR MEALS FOR EACH MEAL TIME. FOR EXAMPLE, MAKING IT PART OF YOUR ROUTINE TO HAVE EGGS FOR BREAKFAST AND A CHICKEN SALAD FOR LUNCH.

STEP 3:
SCHEDULE YOUR TRAINING

Schedule your resistance training and cardio workouts for the upcoming week as outlined in *'Transformation Training'*.

Here is a summary of the points we covered earlier on workout nutrition:

▶ If training during the daytime, time your workout to fall between two of your normal meals.

▶ Leave at least one hour between the pre-workout meal and the start of your workout to avoid stomach upset.

▶ If training first thing in the morning, or at some other point during the day where you have not eaten for more than four to six hours, have a pre-workout snack or schedule a meal for straight after your workout.

AND, DO NOT FORGET...

In addition to scheduling your meals and training, you also need to:

▶ Find time for walks to hit your daily step target.

▶ Update MFP (do this after each meal rather than waiting).

▶ Message your diet partner with a summary of your day.

Keep hold of your completed weekly meal plan sheets as you will be able to spot patterns and trends emerge over time that will help you to learn from the experience.

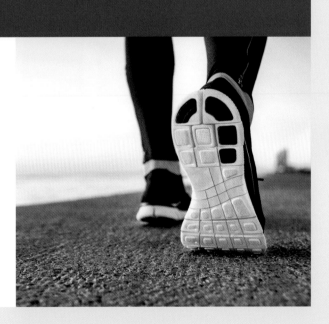

	SUN	MON	TUE	WED	THU	FRI	SAT (REFEED DAY)
6 AM – 8 AM	MEAL 1	MEAL 1	MEAL 1	MEAL 1	MEAL 1	MEAL 1	MEAL 1
8 AM – 10 AM							FORMAL CARDIO
10 AM – 12 NOON	MEAL 2	MEAL 2	MEAL 2	WORK MEAL OUT	MEAL 2	MEAL 2	MEAL 2
12 NOON – 2 PM							
2 PM – 4 PM	MEAL 3	MEAL 3	MEAL 3	MEAL 3	MEAL 3	MEAL 3	MEAL 3
4 PM – 6 PM		RESISTANCE TRAINING	RESISTANCE TRAINING		RESISTANCE TRAINING	RESISTANCE TRAINING	
6 PM – 8 PM	MEAL 4	MEAL 4	MEAL 4	MEAL 4	MEAL 4	MEAL 4	SOCIAL MEAL OUT
8 PM – 10 PM	DIET PARTNER CHECK IN	DIET PARTNER CHECK IN	DIET PARTNER CHECK IN	DIET PARTNER CHECK IN	DIET PARTNER CHECK IN	DIET PARTNER CHECK IN	DIET PARTNER CHECK IN

PROGRESS ASSESSMENT

PROGRESS ASSESSMENT

THE AIM OF THIS SECTION IS TO SHOW YOU HOW TO COMPLETE THE ULTIMATE PERFORMANCE BODY COMPOSITION ASSESSMENT.

There are four parts to the assessment:

- ☐ Bodyweight.

- ☐ Circumference measurements.

- ☐ Progress pictures.

- ☐ Body fat percentage estimate.

We will also explain how to track adherence to your training and meal plan.

Once you have read this guide, make sure to read the *'How to Make Changes'* section to learn how to interpret and respond to your results.

The Importance of a Precision Mindset

When completing the assessment, you must adopt a precision mindset to avoid measurement errors affecting the reliability of your results.

The table below details some of the most common sources of measurement error in body composition assessment.

MEASUREMENT ERROR	EXAMPLE
Inconsistent measurement technique	Measuring your navel circumference at a different level each time.
Faulty measurement instruments	Cloth and fibreglass tape measures can become stretched over time.
Equipment limitations	Bodyweight scales only show how much you have lost or gained, not what you have lost or gained, e.g. fat, muscle, water or food weight.
Measurements difficulties	Attempting to take circumference measurements by yourself.
Changes in environment and time of measurement	Weighing yourself in the morning and evening or taking pictures before and after workouts.
Changes in physiology	Bodyweight fluctuations throughout a women's menstrual cycle due to water retention (and not body fat gain or loss).

The biggest risks of measurement errors are that they can lead you to think that:

▶ You are making progress when you are not (also known as a 'false positive').

▶ You are not making progress when you are (also known as a 'false negative').

False positive results can cause you to lose valuable time as you do not realise that you may need to make changes to start seeing real progress.

False negatives can be equally frustrating, as they make it appear like your hard work is having no impact. They can also prompt you to make a change when you do not need to, like reducing your calorie intake, which makes your diet unnecessarily challenging!

So, how can you avoid measurement errors?

By taking the following actions, which we will guide you through in this section:

▶ Use standardised measurement techniques and procedures.

▶ Use high-quality equipment.

▶ Use more than one assessment method.

▶ Take repeat measurements.

▶ Carefully interpret your results.

BODYWEIGHT

What You Need

- ☐ Digital bodyweight scales.

- ☐ Position the scales on a flat, hard surface, e.g. bathroom tiles, rather than an uneven, soft surface, e.g. carpet.

Frequency and Timing

- ▶ You need a single morning bodyweight reading to create your starting meal plan.

- ▶ During your transformation, aim for seven readings per week and a minimum of three.

- ▶ Weigh yourself first thing in the morning. Make a note of the time and aim to keep this consistent (where possible).

TRAINER TIPS:

If you do not have access to your regular scales, e.g. when travelling, and it is only for a few days, you can either use a different set of scales, e.g. hotel room or wait until you return home to start weighing yourself again.

You will almost always weigh more in the evening than you do in the morning due to added weight from food and drink. This is why we recommend weighing yourself upon waking for the most consistent readings.

Recording the time of measurement can help explain daily fluctuations in your bodyweight. For example, you would most likely be heavier if you weighed yourself at 5 am versus 10 am due to having more undigested food in your stomach (the timing of your last meal can also cause bodyweight fluctuations).

How to Measure

- ▶ Weigh yourself wearing minimal or no clothing, after using the bathroom and before eating or drinking anything.

- ▶ At the end of each week, calculate your weekly average bodyweight. To do this, add up the readings and divide by the total number of days measured.

- ▶ Calculate the percentage change between your latest weekly average bodyweight and the previous week's average. You will be able to do this from the end of week 2, e.g. week 1 vs week 2, week 2 vs week 3, and so on.

- ▶ We recommend searching online for a 'percentage change calculator' to do the maths for you. Enter your old average as the first value, and your new one as the second value.

EXAMPLE BODYWEIGHT READINGS

Day	Week 1 Bodyweight	Week 2 Bodyweight	Week 3 Bodyweight	Week 4 Bodyweight
Day 1	80kg	79.5kg	79.2kg	78.5kg
Day 2	80.5kg	79.4kg	78.9kg	78.4kg
Day 3	80.3kg	79.6kg	79kg	78.6kg
Day 4	80kg	79.4kg	79.1kg	78.3kg
Day 5	79.9kg	79.2kg	79kg	78.1kg
Day 6	79.7kg	79.1kg	78.5kg	78.2kg
Day 7	79.8kg	79.1kg	78.4kg	78.1kg
Average	80kg	79.3kg	78.8kg	78.3kg
% change	-0.88%		-0.63%	

Bodyweight Fluctuations and What They Mean

Bodyweight changes provide valuable feedback, but you need to interpret them carefully.

When the scale moves up or down it only tells you how much you have lost or gained, not what you have lost or gained.

Your bodyweight can fluctuate daily by 1-3% without any change in your current amount of body fat or muscle mass. Daily fluctuations are mainly due to changes in your body's water balance ('water weight') and the amount of food retained in your system at any given time.

The table below details the long list of factors that can cause your bodyweight to fluctuate.

WATER BALANCE	FOOD WEIGHT
Sweat	Bowel movements
Carbohydrate intake	Time of last meal
Sodium intake	Time of weigh-in
Water intake	Refeeds (more food in your system)
Refeeds	
Menstrual cycle	
Stress levels	
Medication	
Illness	

YOUR BODYWEIGHT CAN FLUCTUATE DAILY BY 1-3% WITHOUT ANY CHANGE IN YOUR CURRENT AMOUNT OF BODY FAT OR MUSCLE MASS. DAILY FLUCTUATIONS ARE MAINLY DUE TO CHANGES IN YOUR BODY'S WATER BALANCE ('WATER WEIGHT') AND THE AMOUNT OF FOOD RETAINED IN YOUR SYSTEM AT ANY GIVEN TIME.

To help make sense of scale weight fluctuations, we can use the same '3,500 calorie rule' that you used to create your meal plan. Recall that a single pound of body fat (0.45kg) contains roughly 3,500kcal. Based on this:

▶ To store one pound of body fat, you need to consume at least 3,500kcal more than your maintenance calorie intake.

▶ To lose one pound of body fat, you need to consume at least 3,500kcal less than your maintenance calorie intake.

Weight loss is not a linear process and several weird things will happen to your bodyweight over the course of your transformation.

The images below show how our example client Jenny's bodyweight can fluctuate and how she can use the 3,500kcal test to keep calm when stepping on the scale!

SUDDEN WEIGHT GAIN

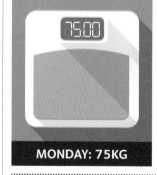
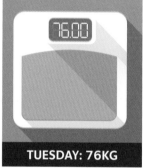

MONDAY: 75KG | **TUESDAY: 76KG**

What Did Not Happen

Jenny's estimated maintenance calorie intake is 2,255kcal. For her to gain a kilogram of body fat overnight, she would have had to have consumed 9,955kcal on Monday. Clearly, this did not happen.

What Might Have Happened

Jenny might have eaten late on Monday night, weighed-in earlier than normal on Tuesday morning or had a refeed on Monday where she ate a lot of carbohydrate and sodium-rich foods, which almost always cause a spike in bodyweight when eaten in large quantities.

WEIGHT LOSS IS NOT A LINEAR PROCESS AND SEVERAL WEIRD THINGS WILL HAPPEN TO YOUR BODYWEIGHT OVER THE COURSE OF YOUR TRANSFORMATION.

SUDDEN WEIGHT LOSS

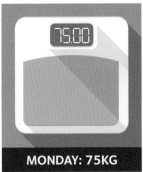 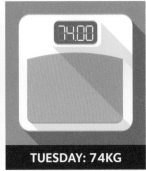

What Did Not Happen

Like how gaining a kilogram of body fat overnight is not possible, Jenny cannot expect to suddenly lose a kilogram overnight.

To do this, she would have had to have eaten nothing all day on Monday and burned an extra 5,445kcal more than she normally does. Again, this clearly did not happen.

What Might Have Happened

Jenny might have survived a stressful period at work, finished a course of medication or entered the stage of her menstrual cycle where her bodyweight is lowest.

LIKE HOW GAINING A KILOGRAM OF BODY FAT OVERNIGHT IS NOT POSSIBLE, JENNY CANNOT EXPECT TO SUDDENLY LOSE A KILOGRAM OVERNIGHT.

SUDDEN WEIGHT LOSS STALL

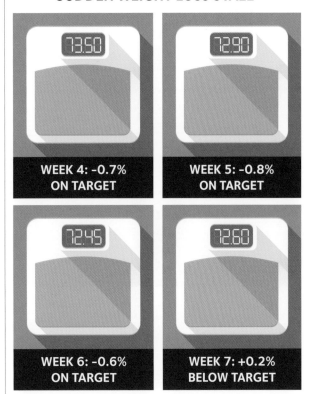

What Did Not Happen

In the above example, the percentage change in Jenny's bodyweight between weeks was on target (-0.5-1% per week) in week 4, 5 and 6, but was below target (less than -0.5%) in week 7.

The body's adaptive response to fat loss occurs over a period of months, not days. So, Jenny's body has not gone into 'starvation mode' and the meal plan and training program that worked in weeks 4-6 should still be effective in week 5.

What Might Have Happened

Jenny's progress may have stalled in week 7 due to random bodyweight fluctuations outside of her control. Alternatively, she may have deviated from her meal plan and not stuck to her nutrition targets as rigorously as normal.

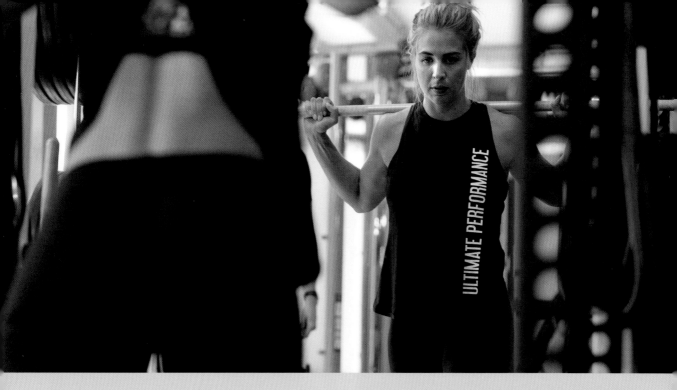

Female Bodyweight Fluctuations

A woman's bodyweight can fluctuate very little or by as much as several pounds over the course of her menstrual cycle – typically peaking before menstruation.

A comprehensive overview of the menstrual cycle is beyond the scope of this book. However, we do recommend tracking your cycle and consulting a medical professional if you have any concerns.

There are several smartphone applications you can use, or you can keep a manual record, recording the first day of your period as '1' and so on.

A WOMAN'S BODYWEIGHT CAN FLUCTUATE VERY LITTLE OR BY AS MUCH AS SEVERAL POUNDS OVER THE COURSE OF HER MENSTRUAL CYCLE – TYPICALLY PEAKING BEFORE MENSTRUATION.

RECOMMENDATIONS

▶ Follow the best practice outlined above when measuring your bodyweight. Try to view your daily weigh-in as data collection and focus on the weekly average.

▶ Use the 3,500kcal test to troubleshoot bodyweight fluctuations. If your bodyweight shoots up overnight, ask yourself, 'did I massively overeat yesterday?', If the answer is no, then you are simply retaining water or have more food in your system than normal.

▶ The best ways to manage water retention are to stay hydrated, eat plenty of vegetables, exercise and be consistent with your diet.

CIRCUMFERENCE MEASUREMENTS

What You Need

☐ Tape measure calibrated in centimetres with millimetre markings. Use the same tape measure every time.

☐ Friend or family member to help take the measurements.

☐ We recommend men wear shorts and no top, and women wear shorts and sports bra.

TRAINER TIPS:

Make sure your tape measure is in good condition. Cloth and fibreglass tape measures can stretch and become twisted over time making it hard to take an accurate measurement.

From experience, the most reliable tape measure is the Lufkin W606PM.

MAKE SURE YOUR TAPE MEASURE IS IN GOOD CONDITION. CLOTH AND FIBREGLASS TAPE MEASURES CAN STRETCH AND BECOME TWISTED OVER TIME MAKING IT HARD TO TAKE AN ACCURATE MEASUREMENT.

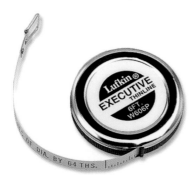

Frequency and Timing

☐ We have highlighted the sites you need to measure on the diagram overleaf, which differ slightly for men and women.

MEN: Measure height, neck and navel at the baseline body composition assessment. After this, continue to measure your navel once per week.

WOMEN: Measure height, neck, natural waist, navel and hips at the baseline body composition assessment. After this, continue to measure your navel and hips once per week.

☐ Record first thing in the morning, after using the bathroom and before eating or drinking anything (where possible).

☐ If measuring later in the day, make a note of the time and number of meals eaten. Aim for a consistent time and always measure before training.

☐ Do not take measurements after training or using a sauna/shower, as exercise, heat and warm water can affect your results.

TRAINER TIPS:

The two sites we are most interested in for ongoing progress assessment are the navel and hips.

Men typically hold most of their body fat on their upper body, specifically around their stomach. In contrast, women tend to carry more body fat on their lower body, specifically on their hips and thighs.

How to Measure

The following instructions are for you to follow when having your measurements taken:

▶ Stand upright with your feet shoulder-width apart and arms hanging by your sides.

▶ Once the tape measure is in position, breathe normally.

The following instructions are for your assistant to follow:

▶ When positioning the tape measure, try to minimise any gaps between the tape and body surface. But, do not hold the tape measure too tight as skin compression produces artificially low readings.

Continuous contact is not always possible on some measurement sites, e.g. across the lower back when measuring the navel.

▶ If measuring over clothing, e.g. shorts, apply enough tension to minimise the effect of the clothing.

▶ Make sure the tape measure is level and not twisted.

▶ When reading the tape measure, your eyes should be at the same level as the tape.

▶ Hold the tape measure in place for a few full breaths and then read the measurement at the end of a normal exhalation.

▶ Record measurements to the nearest 0.1cm, e.g. 85.6cm.

▶ Perform two measurements at each site and calculate the average. To do this, add the measurements together and divide by the total number of readings.

▶ If the two measurements differ by more than 0.5cm, take an extra measurement and calculate the average of the two closest readings.

CIRCUMFERENCE MEASUREMENTS

Site	Measurement 1	Measurement 2	Measurement 3	Average
Height	180cm	Not needed	Not needed	-
Neck	45cm	44.5cm	Not needed	44.8cm
Natural Waist	86cm	86.5cm	Not needed	86.3cm
Navel	89cm	~~87.5cm~~	88.7cm	88.9cm
Hips	92cm	92.4cm	Not needed	92.2cm

TRAINER TIPS:

You should read the measurements at eye level to avoid parallax errors. A parallax error occurs when you read a different value on a measuring device depending on your viewing angle. For example, looking down at your protein shaker and trying to fill it up to 500ml versus holding it at eye level.

Make sure the tape measure is level and not twisted when taking the measurements. From experience, all sites need at least some adjustment.

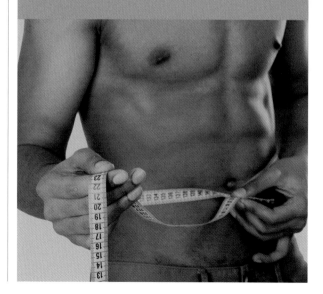

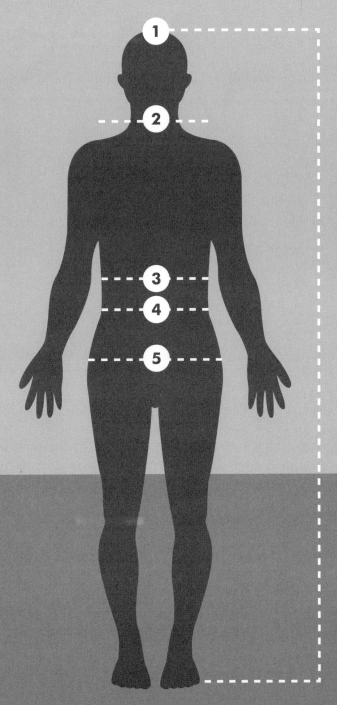

KEY MEASUREMENTS

1 HEIGHT
(without shoes)

2 NECK
(Measure just below
your larynx)

3 NATURAL WAIST
(Measure over the narrowest
part of your waist)

4 NAVEL
(Measure over your
belly button)

5 HIPS
(Measure over the greatest
protrusion of your buttocks
- as viewed from the side).

MEN: Measure height, neck and navel at the baseline body composition assessment. After this, continue to measure your navel once per week.

WOMEN: Measure height, neck, natural waist, navel and hips at the baseline body composition assessment. After this, continue to measure your navel and hips once per week.

PROGRESS PICTURES

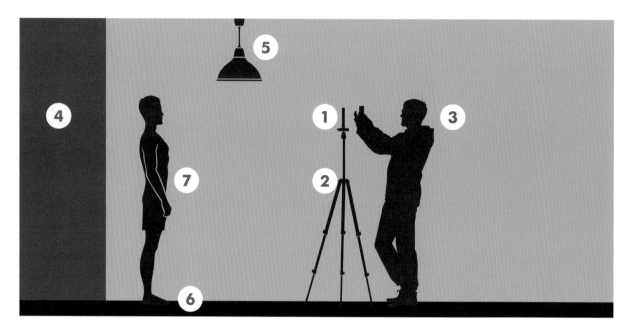

What You Need

1. Smartphone or camera.

2. Smartphone or camera tripod to help ensure consistent height and angle (optional, but relatively inexpensive and greatly improves the quality of pictures).

3. Friend or family member to take the pictures. Alternatively, you can use the self-timer function on your camera (selfies taken in the mirror holding a camera will not do!).

4. Use the same location. Ideally, a clear, white or dark background that is free from any distractions and clutter.

5. Use the same lighting every time. Too bright and it washes all the detail out. Too dark and you will cast shadows that can mask progress.

6. Floor markings (optional).

7. Wear the same clothing every time. We recommend men wear shorts and no top, and women wear shorts and sports bra.

TRAINER TIPS:

Adjust your shorts to around waist height or just below so that they are not holding in body fat. Remember, the pictures are for you to document your progress, not to share with the world!

If you do not have an appropriate space to take your pictures at home, most commercial gyms have studios with blank walls that you can use.

Frequency and Timing

- [ ] Take your first set of pictures at the baseline body composition assessment. After this, retake them every four weeks.

- [ ] Take pictures first thing in the morning, after using the bathroom and before eating or drinking anything (where possible).

- [ ] If taking pictures later in the day, make a note of the time and number of meals eaten. Aim for a consistent time and always take them before training.

TRAINER TIPS:

Taking pictures after a workout can be incredibly motivating, especially towards the end of your transformation. But always take your progress assessment pictures pre-workout.

From experience, four weeks is the average amount of time you need to wait to see significant changes in progress pictures.

You can take progress pictures more frequently, e.g. every two weeks, which gives you an opportunity to practice and an extra source of accountability. But, do not be too disheartened if you cannot see transformational changes each time.

How to Measure

The following instructions are for you to follow when having your pictures taken:

▶ Stand roughly one foot in front of the wall.

▶ Stand upright with your feet shoulder-width apart and arms hanging by your side. Look straight ahead and do not forget to smile!

▶ See the pictures below for examples of the four different poses.

The following instructions are for you or your assistant to follow when setting up to take the pictures:

▶ Set the camera height between chin and eye level.

▶ Position the camera far enough away to include your full body in the picture. You can always zoom in later, but you cannot zoom out!

▶ Keep the phone vertical and not tilted up or down to avoid distorting the pictures.

▶ Take several pictures for each pose, review them to see if they are in focus and retake if needed.

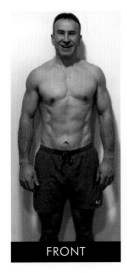
FRONT

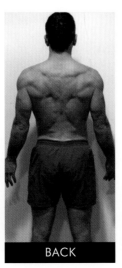
BACK

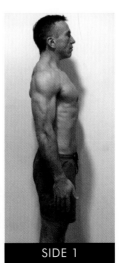
SIDE 1

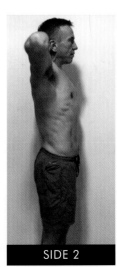
SIDE 2

How to Compare Your Progress Pictures

After each progress picture update, you need to compare the latest pictures to your previous ones to assess your progress.

To do this, you will need to download a photo collage application to your smartphone or computer. Search your mobile's app store or online for 'free photo collage maker'.

Like MFP, we cannot give detailed instructions on how to use a specific application. But, here are some guidelines to follow when creating collages:

▶ If you keep the camera height and angle consistent each time, then the pictures should fit together without needing much adjustment.

▶ Take your time to make sure the pictures are the same size and line up. Position the pictures so that your shoulders are level and zoom in and out until your head is the same size in each picture.

▶ Keep the pictures organised by date in a folder on your laptop or smartphone.

▶ Record in your progress tracker if you can see a visible change between the pictures.

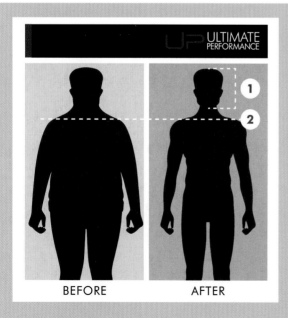

CONSISTENCY IS KEY

1 The head should be the same size.

2 Shoulders should be level.

BODY FAT PERCENTAGE

What is Body Fat Percentage?

Your body fat percentage is the weight of all the fat on your body (fat mass) divided by your total bodyweight. For example, if you weigh 80kg and have 10kg of body fat, your body fat percentage is 12.5%.

Why Measure Your Body Fat Percentage?

Measuring your body fat percentage allows you to track your fat loss progress over time. You can also use it to calculate how much lean body mass (LBM) you have, which is the total weight of your body minus all your fat mass.

A common misunderstanding is that LBM only refers to muscle, when in fact it describes everything in your body apart from body fat. So, in addition to muscle, it also includes things like your organs, bones, skin, body water and food weight.

When creating your meal plan, you will base your calculations on how much LBM you have, rather than total bodyweight.

This distinction is important because body fat and LBM do not have the same energy or nutrient requirements.

A COMMON MISUNDERSTANDING IS THAT LBM ONLY REFERS TO MUSCLE, WHEN IN FACT IT DESCRIBES EVERYTHING IN YOUR BODY APART FROM BODY FAT. SO, IN ADDITION TO MUSCLE, IT ALSO INCLUDES THINGS LIKE YOUR ORGANS, BONES, SKIN, BODY WATER AND FOOD WEIGHT.

Each day your body burns roughly 12kcal per pound maintaining its current amount of LBM. In contrast, although your fat cells are more than just passive storage sites for fat and perform several essential functions, like hormone production, they have a relatively low maintenance cost of 2kcal per pound.

If you are relatively lean, this is not really an issue. For example, if you weigh 80kg and have 10% body fat, then whether you decide to use 80kg or 72kg (your LBM) to create your meal plan will not make a big difference.

However, if you carry a lot more body fat (upwards of 30%), then calculating your calorie requirements based on your total bodyweight will overestimate how many calories you need.

This also applies to other nutrition targets that we traditionally set relative to bodyweight, such as protein. The primary role of protein is structural which means that your body uses it to build and repair components of your LBM such as muscle.

As a result, it makes sense to set your protein target relative to how much LBM you have, rather than body fat, which does not require large amounts of protein.

How to Measure Your Body Fat Percentage

The only way to directly measure your body fat is via cadaver analysis (dissection of a dead human body), which has some obvious practical limitations.

All other methods of body fat testing only estimate how much body fat you have.

An in-depth review of every available body fat assessment tool is beyond the scope of this book, but we have provided a brief overview of the most commonly available.

Each body fat assessment tool is based on a different set of assumptions, and you cannot compare your results between them.

SKINFOLD CALIPER TESTING

The skinfold caliper technique is based on the assumption that there is a relationship between the thickness of skinfolds (which includes the 'pinchable' subcutaneous fat just beneath your skin) at various sites around your body and your total body fat.

Of all the available options, skinfold testing is the most cost-effective and practical method of body fat assessment available to personal trainers.

The primary limitation of skinfold calipers is that measurement reliability depends on the skill and experience level of the operator. Measuring just 1cm away from a defined measurement site produces significant differences in measurement values.

As a result, we do not recommend using skinfold testing unless you have access to a personal trainer who has a relevant qualification and experience at taking measurements.

HIGH-TECH METHODS: DUAL ENERGY X-RAY ABSORPTIOMETRY (DXA) AND HYDROSTATIC WEIGHING

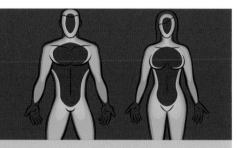

Two examples of more high-tech options are dual-energy x-ray absorptiometry (DXA) and hydrostatic weighing.

A DXA scan is a special type of x-ray that works by sending low-dose x-rays through your body and measuring the absorption rates of different body tissues. The rationale is that body fat and LBM have different absorption properties which allows them to be isolated and measured.

Hydrostatic weighing (also known as underwater weighing) involves comparing your dry weight on land to your underwater weight. Components of LBM like bone and muscle are denser than water whereas fat is

less dense. As a result, if two people weigh the same on dry land but one has more body fat, the fatter person will weigh less underwater.

Put simply, fat floats and muscle sinks!

While DXA and hydrostatic weighing may be more accurate than some low-tech options, they are expensive and impractical (require you to visit a research laboratory or clinic) for the purposes of creating a meal plan and monitoring short-term changes in your body composition.

However, you may decide to get one at the start and end of your transformation, or annually, if you want to learn more about your body composition.

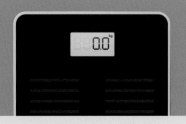

YOUR BATHROOM SCALES

Bioelectrical impedance (BIA) is the technical name for the technology found in bodyweight scales that also estimate your body fat percentage.

It works by sending a small electrical signal through your body and measuring the resistance of different body tissues to the signal.

Body fat can then be estimated based on the fact that the current flows more easily through parts of your body that have high water contents, e.g. muscle and blood, than it does those with low water contents, e.g. bone or fat.

A big problem with BIA devices is that they are incredibly sensitive to changes in your body's water balance. Exercise, food, drink and going to the

bathroom can all affect the reliability of your results.

Overall, there is limited research to support the accuracy of consumer-grade devices, so we recommend only using your scales to weigh yourself.

A BIG PROBLEM WITH BIA DEVICES IS THAT THEY ARE INCREDIBLY SENSITIVE TO CHANGES IN YOUR BODY'S WATER BALANCE. EXERCISE, FOOD, DRINK AND GOING TO THE BATHROOM CAN ALL AFFECT THE RELIABILITY OF YOUR RESULTS.

TAPE MEASUREMENTS

The tape measurement method involves measuring the circumference of various sites around your body and inputting the results into one of several prediction equations.

One of the most popular equations was developed by the U.S. Navy who needed a quick, inexpensive and reasonably accurate method of assessing the body composition of their personnel.

The Navy developed individual equations for men and women, which take into account gender differences in body fat distribution.

The major advantages of the tape measurement method are that it is simple to perform and only requires a tape measure.

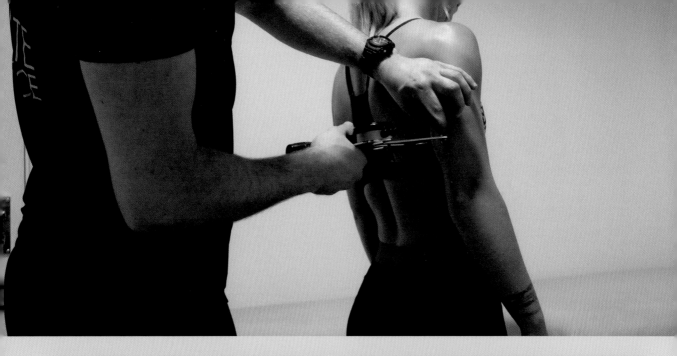

RECOMMENDATIONS

At Ultimate Performance, we measure our client's body fat percentage using skinfold calipers, but we appreciate that not everybody has access to this method of testing.

If this is the case, we recommend using the **Navy equation.**

Admittedly, the Navy equation is not accurate enough to identify your exact body fat percentage, for example, whether you are 16% or 17% body fat, but it can help narrow it down to a relatively tight range.

Once you have used the equation to help set up your starting meal plan, you do not need to (but still can) re-calculate your body fat percentage throughout your transformation.

How to Use the Navy Method

1. MEN: Following the best practice for taking tape measurements outlined earlier, measure your navel, neck and height.

---

2. WOMEN: Following the best practice for taking tape measurements outlined earlier, measure your natural waist, hips, neck and height.

---

3. The equations require some relatively complex maths, so we have provided a Navy body fat calculator on our website, www.upfitness.com

ADHERENCE

What is Adherence?

Adherence is a measure of how closely you follow the nutrition and training guidelines that make up your transformation program.

A lack of adherence, also known as non-compliance, refers to situations where you deviate from one or more parts of the program.

There are two types of non-compliance:

▶ **Conscious non-compliance:** Refers to situations where you know that you have deviated from the program. For example, intentionally overeating, missing a workout or not taking enough steps.

▶ **Unconscious non-compliance:** Refers to situations where you think you are following the program, but actually are not. For example, underestimating the calories in a restaurant meal or misinterpreting an instruction.

How to Track Dietary Adherence

▶ At the end of each day, make a note of your total calorie and protein intake.

▶ Make a note next to any day where you at least partially guesstimated your intake, e.g. dining out.

▶ At the end of each week, calculate your average calorie and protein intake. To do this, add up each day's totals and divide by the total number of days.

▶ Once you have calculated your weekly averages, compare them to your targets and see if they fall within the target ranges, e.g. +/– 50kcal and +/–10g protein.

DIETARY ADHERENCE

Day	Calories	Protein	Notes
1	2,050kcal	180g	
2	2,085kcal	170g	
3	2,100kcal	185g	
4	2,042kcal	175g	Restaurant lunch, approx 850kcal
5	1,980kcal	160g	
6	2,150kcal	180g	
7	2,050kcal	185g	
Average	2,065kcal	176g	

How to Track Training Adherence

▶ At the end of each week, make a note of how many of the scheduled resistance training and formal cardio workouts you completed.

▶ At the end of each week, calculate your average daily steps. To do this, add up each day's step count and divide by the total number of days.

TRAINING ADHERENCE

Day	Training Summary
1	10,000 steps + Resistance training
2	10,500 steps
3	11,000 steps + Resistance training
4	9,500 steps
5	13,000 steps + Resistance training
6	12,500 steps + Formal cardio
7	12,000 steps
Average	**11,214 steps**

ULTIMATE PERFORMANCE PROGRESS TRACKER

The 'Ultimate Performance Progress Tracker' is the tool we use to document a client's progress throughout their transformation. We will explain how to use the tracker in the next section, *How to Make Changes*.

	BASELINE	WEEK 1	WEEK 2	WEEK 3	WEEK 4
BODYWEIGHT					
Bodyweight Average	kg	kg	kg	kg	kg
% Change	–	–	%	%	%
CIRCUMFERENCE MEASUREMENTS					
Naval Circumference	cm	cm	cm	cm	cm
Hip Circumference	cm	cm	cm	cm	cm
ADHERENCE					
Kcal Average	–	kcal	kcal	kcal	kcal
Protein Average	–	g	g	g	g
Step Average	–	steps	steps	steps	steps
Resistance Training Workouts Completed	–	/	/	/	/
Formal Cardio Workouts Completed	–	/	/	/	/
PROGRESS PICTURES					
Visible Change in Pictures?	Before Pics	–	Optional Yes / No	–	Yes / No

Note: We have included an example completed tracker on the next page with summary notes on how to record your body composition assessment.

	WEEK 6	WEEK 7	WEEK 8	WEEK 9	WEEK 10	WEEK 11	WEEK 12
kg	kg	kg	kg	kg	kg	kg	kg
%	%	%	%	%	%	%	%
m	cm	cm	cm	cm	cm	cm	cm
m	cm	cm	cm	cm	cm	cm	cm
cal	kcal	kcal	kcal	kcal	kcal	kcal	kcal
g	g	g	g	g	g	g	g
os	steps	steps	steps	steps	steps	steps	steps
/	/	/	/	/	/	/	/
/	/	/	/	/	/	/	/
	Optional Yes / No	–	Yes / No	–	Optional Yes / No	–	After Pics

Baseline:
Record details of your baseline body composition assessment here.

You only need to record a single morning bodyweight reading for your baseline assessment.

We have not included body fat, height or neck and natural waist circumferences in the tracker as you only need to measure these once to help create your starting meal plan.

Bodyweight:
Weigh yourself 3-7 mornings per week and calculate the weekly average and % change between weeks.

Circumference Measurements:
Retake your circumference measurements at the end of each week.

	BASELINE	WEEK 1	WEEK 2	WEEK 3	WEEK 4	WEEK 5	WEEK 6	WEEK 7	WEEK 8	WEEK 9	WEEK 10	WEEK 11	WEEK 12
BODYWEIGHT													
Bodyweight Average	72.5 kg	71.8 kg	71.2 kg	70.7 kg	70.1 kg	69.6 kg	69.3 kg	68.8 kg	68.1 kg	67.7 kg	67.2 kg	66.6 kg	66.2 kg
% Change	–	–	-0.84 %	-0.71 %	-0.86 %	-0.72 %	-0.43 %	-0.73 %	-1.03 %	-0.59 %	-0.74 %	-0.90 %	-0.60 %
CIRCUMFERENCE MEASUREMENTS													
Naval Circumference	72.9 cm	71.5 cm	70 cm	68.9 cm	67.8 cm	67.2 cm	66.5 cm	66.3 cm	66.1 cm	66 cm	65.9 cm	65.7 cm	65.4 cm
Hip Circumference	87.5 cm	85.7 cm	84 cm	82.7 cm	81.4 cm	80.6 cm	79.8 cm	79.6 cm	79.3 cm	79.2 cm	79.1 cm	78.8 cm	78.5 cm
ADHERENCE													
Kcal Average	–	1,850 kcal	1,800 kcal	1,830 kcal	1,790 kcal	1,820 kcal	1,760 kcal	1,850 kcal	1,810 kcal	1,840 kcal	1,870 kcal	1,900 kcal	1,850 kcal
Protein Average	–	150 g	155 g	140 g	150 g	145 g	150 g	160 g	155 g	165 g	145 g	155 g	150 g
Step Average	–	10,500	11,040	11,500	12,060	10,900	11,400	13,400	12,540	11,880	11,420	10,900	11,200
Resistance Training Workouts Completed	–	4/4	4/4	4/4	4/4	4/4	4/4	4/4	4/4	4/4	4/4	4/4	4/4
Formal Cardio Workouts Completed	–	1/1	1/1	1/1	1/1	1/1	1/1	1/1	1/1	1/1	1/1	1/1	1/1
PROGRESS PICTURES													
Visible Change in Pictures?	Before Pics	–	Optional Yes / No	–	Yes / No	–	Optional Yes / No	–	Yes / No	–	Optional Yes / No	–	After Pics

Dietary Adherence:
Record your protein and calorie intake daily and calculate the weekly average.

Training Adherence:
Record how many of your scheduled training and formal cardio workouts you completed.

Progress Pictures:
Retake every 2-4 weeks, create a collage and note if you can see a visible change between the pictures.

HOW TO
MAKE CHANGES

WHY YOU NEED TO MAKE CHANGES

NOW THAT WE HAVE REVIEWED HOW TO PERFORM THE BODY COMPOSITION ASSESSMENT, THE NEXT STEP IS TO EXPLAIN HOW TO RESPOND TO YOUR RESULTS.

The first issue to address here are the potential reasons why you may, at some point, need to make a change to your transformation program.

NEED FOR CHANGE #1:
REFINE YOUR STARTING MEAL PLAN

The calculations you completed to create your starting meal plan are estimates based on scientific research findings and textbook theory that are not specific to you as an individual.

As a result, you may need to adjust your nutrition targets in the early stages of your transformation to either start seeing or increase the rate of progress.

While we cannot rule this out entirely, we have made every effort to minimise the potential for error by:

▶ Basing the meal plan calculations on LBM, rather than total bodyweight.

▶ Applying a conservative activity multiplier.

▶ Using a relatively large calorie deficit.

TRUE FAT LOSS PLATEAUS HAPPEN OVER A LOT LONGER TIME FRAME AND IN RESPONSE TO SUBSTANTIAL WEIGHT LOSS (UPWARDS OF 10% OF YOUR TOTAL BODYWEIGHT).

NEED FOR CHANGE #2:
FAT LOSS PLATEAUS

Even if there is no need to change your starting meal plan, you should expect the rate of progress that is possible with your initial calorie target to slow down over time.

This makes sense, as a smaller body naturally requires less energy. If you subtract 10kg from your current bodyweight and redo the meal plan calculations, you will get a lower calorie target. You also need to take into account the metabolic adaptations we discussed when reviewing the rationale for refeeds.

However, it is highly unlikely that a calorie intake capable of producing fat loss in the first few weeks of your transformation will no longer be effective in week 12.

True fat loss plateaus happen over a lot longer time frame and in response to substantial weight loss (upwards of 10% of your total bodyweight).

In fact, a lot of you reading this will go the full 12 weeks without making any changes. This is often the case when only dieting for short periods, which in the big picture, 12 weeks is.

Still, even if a genuine plateau has not occurred, you may decide to make a change to increase the rate of fat loss.

WHEN NOT TO MAKE A CHANGE

Before making any changes to your program in response to a lack of progress, you must undertake an honest assessment of your adherence, i.e. how closely have you been following the program?

The number one cause of fat loss plateaus is a lack of adherence.

Many people either stop following diets (conscious non-compliance - recall the 'New Year dieters' discussed earlier) or are unaware that they are making mistakes that compromise their progress (unconscious non-compliance).

In such cases, you may still need to make a change. But, the change may be to try and improve adherence, rather than to cut calories further or increase training volume.

THE PROGRESS REVIEW SYSTEM

——

WE HAVE SUMMARISED THE BODY COMPOSITION ASSESSMENT AND REVIEW PROCESS INTO THREE KEY STEPS AND WILL GUIDE YOU THROUGH EACH ONE IN DETAIL.

Simply follow along step-by-step to see what changes (if any) you need to make at various stages of your transformation.

STEP 1:
COMPLETE PROGRESS CHECK-IN

Before starting, download a copy of the Ultimate Performance Progress Tracker from our website, www.upfitness.com.

Schedule time at the end of each week of your transformation to perform the following progress check-in:

▶ Calculate weekly average bodyweight and percentage change between weeks.

▶ Retake circumference measurements.

▶ Calculate weekly calorie, protein and step averages.

▶ Record how many of your scheduled workouts you completed.

▶ Take progress pictures if due.

Update your progress tracker with details of the assessment and move on to step 2.

STEP 2:
REVIEW YOUR PROGRESS

Although you will perform the progress check in at the end of week 1, you will not have enough data to review your progress until the end of week 2.

At this point, you can calculate the percentage change in bodyweight between weeks for the first time.

We use changes in bodyweight as the main measure of progress, because:

▶ Spotting early changes in progress pictures requires a 'coach's eye' and most people struggle to objectively assess their own pictures.

▶ Circumference measurements are deceptively tricky to take and there is a risk that measurement error will bias your results.

▶ Most people do not have access to an accurate method of body fat testing.

The aim throughout your transformation is to lose on average between 0.5-1% of your total bodyweight per week.

Here are the possible scenarios you will face when reviewing your progress at the end of each week (starting from week 2) and the recommended actions:

On Target:
Average Bodyweight Dropped by 0.5-1%.

If you are on target, keep up the good work, and reassess at the next progress check in.

Above Target:
Average Bodyweight Dropped by More Than 1%.

If you are above target, ask yourself the following question:

"Am I consistently struggling with hunger and energy levels?"

A simple tip to help distinguish between a craving for food (often triggered by boredom or habit!) and physical hunger is to ask yourself, *'am I hungry enough to eat a plate of broccoli (or least favourite food here)?'.*

If hunger and energy levels are not a problem, carry on and reassess at next check-in.

However, if you are struggling with hunger and energy levels, you should:

▶ Double check that you completed the meal plan calculations correctly and have not set your calorie target too low.

▶ Reread the serving size FAQs to make sure you are not unintentionally undereating, e.g. mistaking 100g of chicken for 100g of protein.

▶ Follow the recommended activity levels and do not attempt to do extra work, e.g. performing extra formal cardio workouts.

If the above points do not address the issue, increase your calorie target, which we will show you how to do in step 3.

Below Target:
Average Bodyweight Dropped by Less Than 0.5% for the First Time.

If you are below target, but were on or above target at the previous week's check-in, the first thing to check for is non-compliance.

Conscious Non-compliance

You can test for conscious non-compliance by reviewing your dietary and training adherence:

▶ Did you meet your calorie target within +/- 50kcal and protein target within +/- 10g? Yes/No

▶ Did you complete all scheduled resistance training and formal cardio workouts? Yes/No

▶ Did you meet your daily average step target? Yes/No

If the answer is no to any of the above, refocus on meeting your targets and reassess at the next check-in.

Unconscious Non-compliance

If you are confident that you have been fully compliant, the next step is to check for unconscious non-compliance.

An experienced personal trainer can spot certain warning signs, such as dining out frequently, but it can be difficult to check yourself, as by definition, you are unaware that there is an issue!

The best way to test for unconscious non-compliance is to aim for the 'perfect week', where you make every effort to follow the program to the letter.

Here are some recommended actions you can take to rule out unconscious non-compliance:

▶ Set time aside to write your meal plan for the upcoming week in advance.

▶ Limit dining out and prepare most of your own meals.

▶ Reread the serving size FAQs.

▶ Make sure you record everything in MFP.

Circumference Measurements and Progress Pictures

A final check you can make is to review your circumference measurements and progress pictures.

Unlike bodyweight, there are no target rates of progress to aim for. Instead, we simply want to see a downward trend in measurements over time and for you to look visibly leaner in each set of progress pictures.

If you were on or above target at the previous week's check in, look leaner since starting, and your measurements have dropped, the plateau is most likely a temporary stall caused by one or a combination of bodyweight fluctuations and non-compliance.

Do not make any changes, aim for the 'perfect week' and reassess at the next progress check-in.

Below Target:
Average Bodyweight Dropped by Less Than 0.5% for Two Consecutive Weeks.

If you are below target for two consecutive weeks and are confident that you are following the program, reduce your calorie target, which we will show you how to do in step 3.

FEMALE BODYWEIGHT FLUCTUATIONS

From experience, temporary weight loss stalls are more common in women due to bodyweight fluctuations throughout the menstrual cycle. As a result, women need to be more careful when reviewing their progress and deciding whether to make a change.

If one of the below target results occurred in the final week of your menstrual cycle, discount this week and delay making any changes for another week.

For example, if you were below target for two consecutive weeks, but the second week was the final week of your cycle, only make a change if the following week is also below target.

STEP 3:
MAKE CHANGES

As you have just learned, there are two possible scenarios that may arise during your transformation that will require you to make a change to your nutrition targets:

▶ You need to increase calories, because you are progressing above target and struggling with hunger and energy levels.

▶ You need to decrease calories, because you have progressed below target for two consecutive progress check-ins.

How to Increase Calories

▶ Increase your daily calorie target by 5%. For example, 1,500kcal becomes 1,575kcal (1,500 x 1.05), 2,000kcal becomes 2,100kcal (2,000 x 1.05), and so on.

▶ Once you have calculated your revised calorie target, return to the macronutrient calculations section (p.39) and follow the steps to work out your new targets. You can take this opportunity to make adjustments to all three macronutrient targets within the recommended guidelines.

▶ Do not increase the refeed calorie target.

How to Decrease Calories

▶ Decrease your calorie target by 10%. For example, 1,500kcal becomes 1,350kcal (1,500 x 0.9), 2,000kcal becomes 1,800kcal (2,000 x 0.9), and so on.

▶ Once you have calculated your revised calorie target, return to the macronutrient calculations section (p.39) and follow the steps to work out your new targets. You can take this opportunity to make adjustments to all three macronutrient targets within the recommended guidelines.

▶ Do not decrease the refeed calorie target.

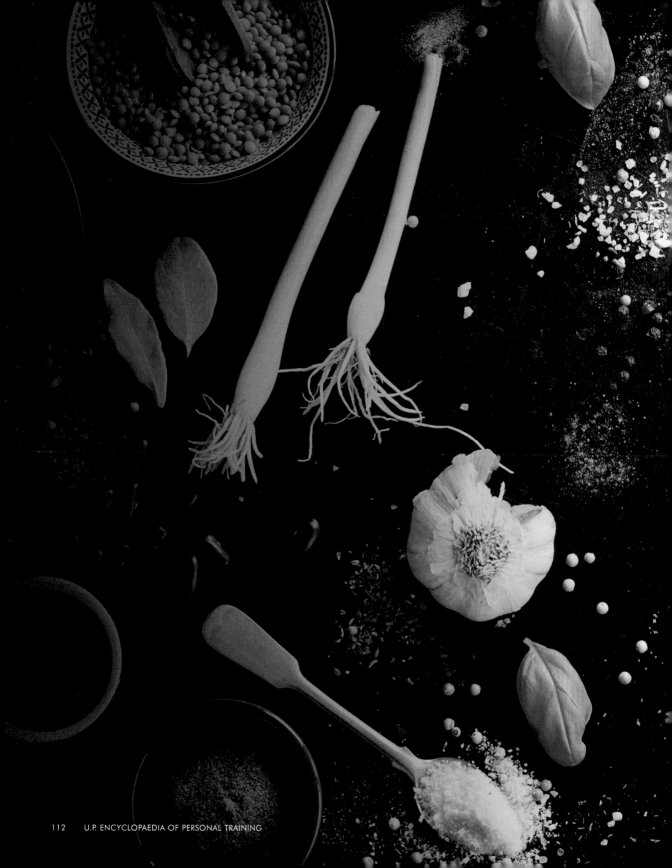

TRANSFORMATION RECIPES

Breakfasts

Low-Carb Main Meals

High-Carb Main Meals

Vegetables and Salads

Refeed Inspiration

TRANSFORMATION RECIPES

By now you should know your transformation numbers and the transformation foods we recommend building your meal plan around.

This section will show you how to combine individual foods into meals that are easy to make, fit with your nutrition targets and taste delicious!

Start with the Basics

Unless you are an experienced cook, we recommend starting with a simple approach to cooking.

Familiarise yourself with the different options in the transformation food tables and practice combining them into simple meals.

Select a protein source, fat source and carbohydrate source and use basic cooking methods like baking, stir-frying, steaming and boiling.

Once you have learned how to prepare meals that meet your nutrition targets, you can start to be more adventurous and experiment with different ingredients and flavour combinations.

Even if you are a competent cook, it helps to have some convenient go-to meals for when you are short on time, for example, busy weekdays.

If you do see a recipe that you would like to try, perhaps the best time to attempt it is on the weekend when you will have more time to prepare and enjoy the meal.

You do not have to use the transformation recipes. In fact, some of our clients prefer to keep their meals plain and simple. If you meet your nutrition targets and stick to the recommended foods, you will get the same results regardless of whether you follow the recipes or not.

How to Follow the Recipes

▶ On days where you want to include a recipe in your meal plan, start by selecting the recipe in advance and then work out how much of your daily food intake this takes up. You can then plan how to spread the remainder of your calories over the rest of the day.

▶ We have written almost all recipes to serve one person, provide 20-50g of protein and total no more than 500 kcal.

▶ If you are cooking for multiple people or batch cooking for yourself, multiply the serving sizes to match your requirements.

▶ All ingredient weights refer to the uncooked weight unless stated otherwise.

▶ Each recipe has a nutrition overview that details the macronutrient and calorie content per serving. Use this as an indicator only and always use the values listed on your product's nutrition label.

You do not have to follow the recipes rigidly and can make certain changes without affecting the outcome. For example,

1. Changing serving sizes for protein, fat and carbohydrate sources to meet your nutrition targets.

2. Swapping out ingredients to match personal taste preferences.

BREAKFASTS

How to Make an Omelette

Smoked Salmon and Dill Omelette

Chicken, Bacon and Tomato Omelette

How to Make Poached Eggs

Poached Eggs with Ham
and Tomato

Poached Eggs with Sourdough
and Avocado

How to Make Pancakes

U.P. Chocotrients Pancakes

Protein Shakes

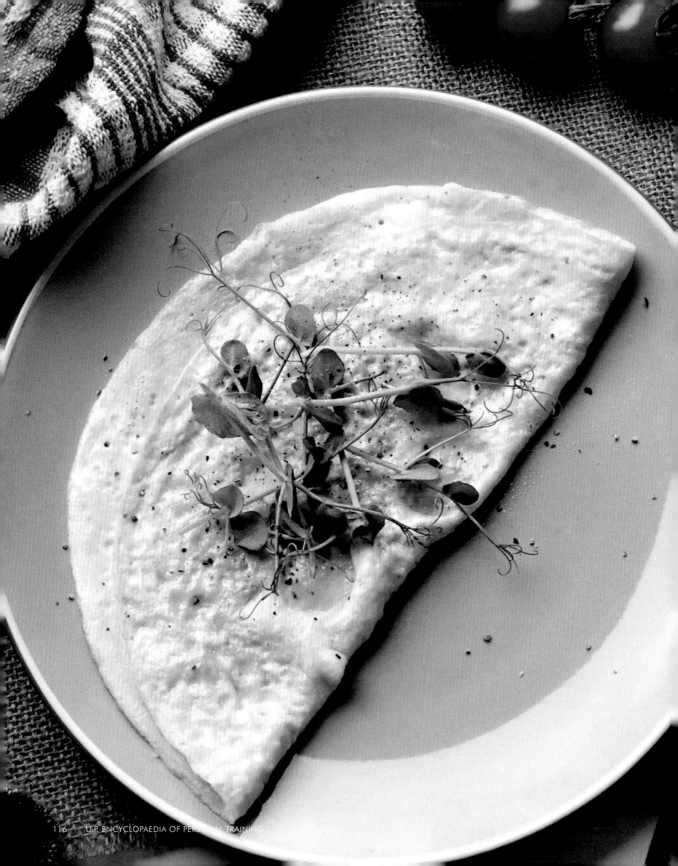

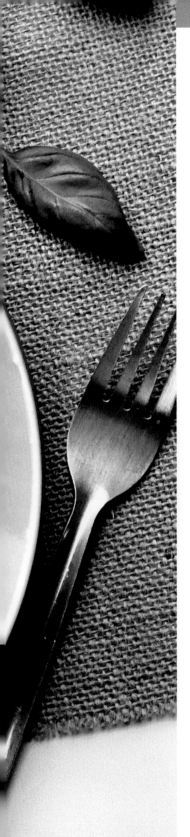

BREAKFASTS

—

HOW TO MAKE AN OMELETTE

PREP TIME: Under 10 mins.
COOK TIME: Under 10 mins.

CALORIES	PROTEIN	FAT	CARBS
150 kCal	15 g	10 g	0 g

EQUIPMENT

- Mixing bowl.
- Whisk or fork.
- Large non-stick frying pan.
- Spatula.

INGREDIENTS

- 2 medium whole eggs.
- Sea salt and black pepper.
- Low-calorie cooking spray.

METHOD

1. Crack the eggs into a mixing bowl and whisk thoroughly. Season with sea salt and black pepper.

2. Place a frying pan lightly coated with low-calorie cooking spray over medium-high heat. Pour the eggs into the pan (if the eggs do not reach the edges, tilt the pan to correct).

3. Remove the pan from the heat when the sides of the omelette start to solidify and the centre begins to bubble.

4. Place the pan under a hot grill for 2 minutes to gently brown the top.

5. Use the spatula to work around the edges of the omelette to check that there are no stubborn areas that have become stuck to the pan.

6. Gently tilt the pan and allow the omelette to slide onto your plate.

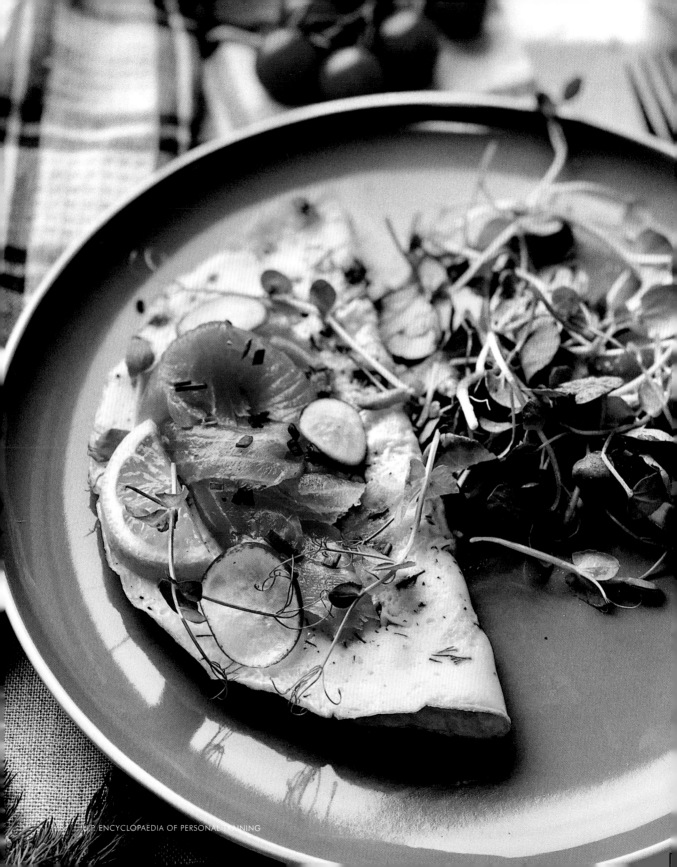

BREAKFASTS

SMOKED SALMON AND DILL OMELETTE

PREP TIME: Under 10 mins.
COOK TIME: Under 10 mins.

CALORIES	PROTEIN	FAT	CARBS
340 kCal	35 g	20 g	0 g

EQUIPMENT

- Digital food scales.
- Mixing bowl.
- Whisk or fork.
- Large non-stick frying pan.
- Spatula.

INGREDIENTS

- 2 medium whole eggs.
- Low-calorie cooking spray.
- 1 tsp chopped fresh dill leaves.

Serve with:

- 50g watercress.
- 100g smoked salmon.
- Cracked black pepper.
- 1 tsp lemon juice (fresh lemon wedge or bottled lemon juice).
- Vegetables of choice - see transformation food tables.

METHOD

1. Start to prepare your omelette following the *'Basic Omelette'* method.

2. While the omelette cooks, sprinkle on the fresh dill so that it sinks into the eggs.

3. Once cooked, lay the omelette flat on your plate and top with watercress.

4. Add the smoked salmon and finish with cracked black pepper and lemon juice.

5. Serve along with any extra vegetables of your choice.

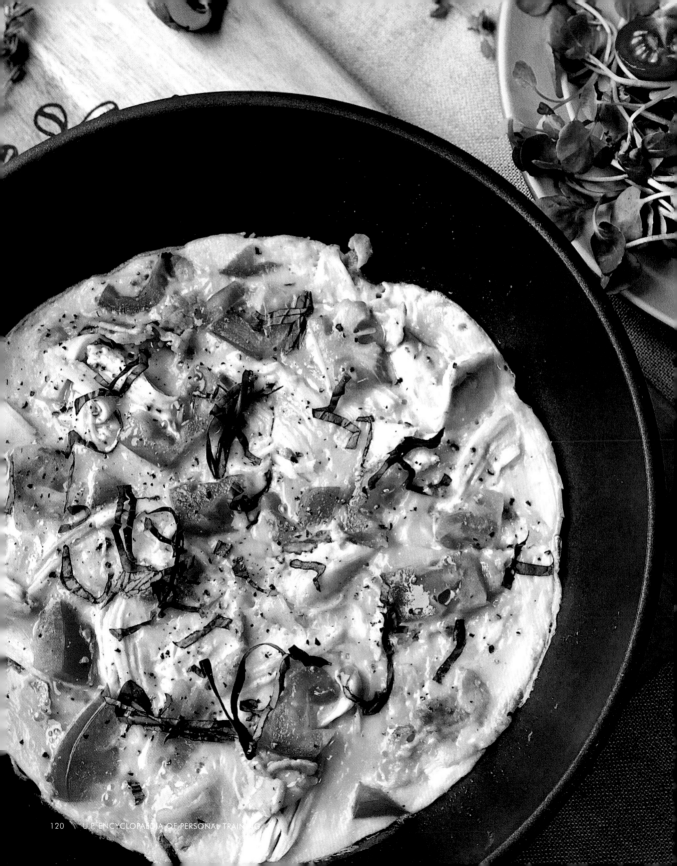

BREAKFASTS

CHICKEN, BACON AND TOMATO OMELETTE

PREP TIME: Under 10 mins.
COOK TIME: Under 30 mins.

CALORIES	PROTEIN	FAT	CARBS
295 kCal	40 g	15 g	0 g

EQUIPMENT

- Digital food scales.
- Mixing bowl.
- Whisk or fork.
- Large non-stick frying pan.
- Baking tray.
- Grill pan.
- Spatula.

INGREDIENTS

- 100g chicken breast.
- 2 medium whole eggs.
- Low-calorie cooking spray.
- 2 bacon slices.
- 1 tomato, diced.
- 1 tsp shredded basil.

Serve with:

- 50g spinach.
- Vegetables of choice - see transformation food tables.

METHOD

1. Preheat your oven to 200°C (fan 180°C/gas mark 6).

2. Roast the chicken breast on a baking tray until cooked through.

3. Remove the cooked chicken from the oven and allow to cool, then use 2 forks (or your fingers) to tear the chicken into thin strips.

4. Prepare the bacon by grilling under a high heat until crispy, then slice into thin strips.

5. Start to prepare your omelette following the *'Basic Omelette'* method.

6. Add the chicken, bacon and tomato to the omelette while the egg mix is still runny. Sprinkle the basil over the omelette.

7. Once cooked, lay the omelette flat on your plate and serve with spinach and any extra vegetables of your choice.

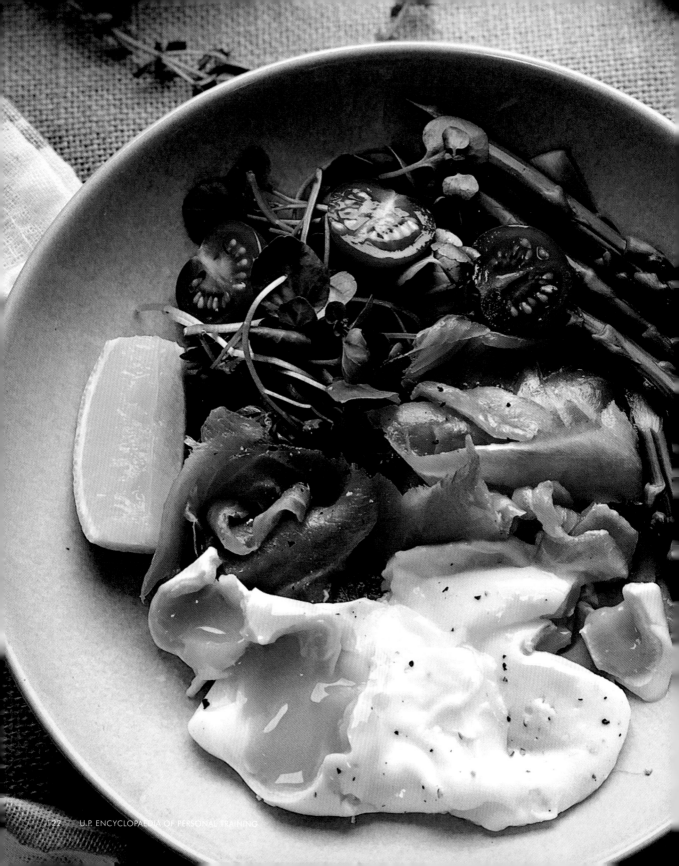

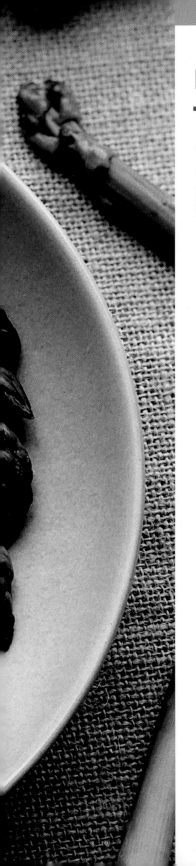

BREAKFASTS

HOW TO MAKE POACHED EGGS

PREP TIME: Under 10 mins.
COOK TIME: Under 10 mins.

CALORIES	PROTEIN	FAT	CARBS
150 kCal	15 g	10 g	0 g

EQUIPMENT

- Large non-stick saucepan with a lid.
- Slotted spoon.

INGREDIENTS

- 1 tsp white wine vinegar.
- 2 medium whole eggs.

METHOD

1. Fill a saucepan with water and add the white wine vinegar. Cover with a lid and bring to the boil.

2. Remove the lid and reduce the heat to bring the water to a gentle simmer.

3. Gently crack the eggs into the pan, close to the surface of the water. Leave them to simmer for 3-4 minutes until they float to the surface.

4. Check if the eggs are ready to serve (the exterior should be firm but not watery).

5. Once cooked, use the slotted spoon to remove the eggs from the water and serve as desired.

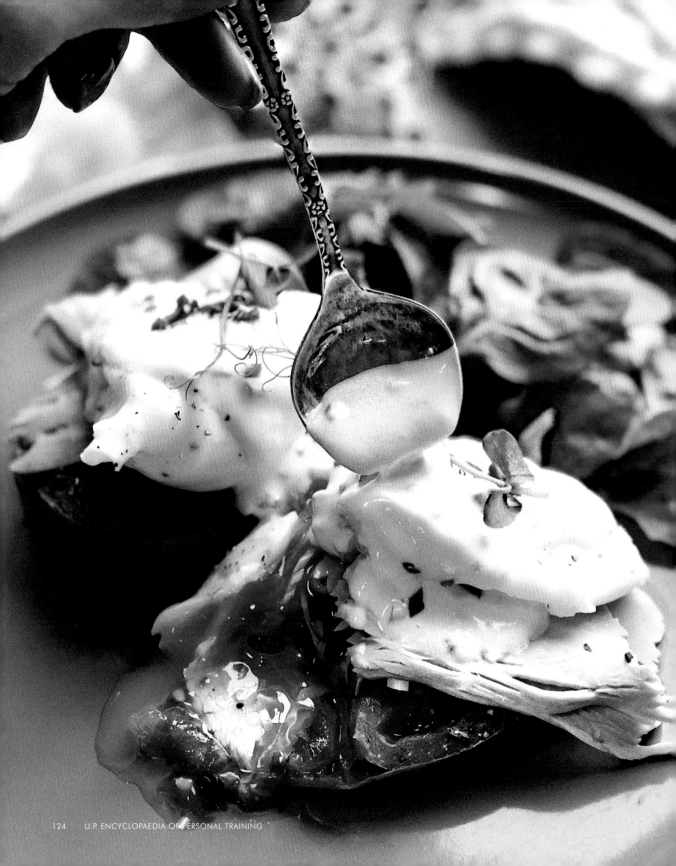

BREAKFASTS

POACHED EGGS WITH HAM AND TOMATO

PREP TIME: Under 10 mins.
COOK TIME: Under 10 mins.

CALORIES	PROTEIN	FAT	CARBS
320 kCal	30 g	20 g	5 g

EQUIPMENT

- Digital food scales.
- Grill pan.
- Large non-stick saucepan with a lid.
- Slotted spoon.
- Baking tray.
- Small non-stick saucepan.

INGREDIENTS

- 2 medium whole eggs.
- 1 tsp white wine vinegar.

For the sauce:
- 50g 0% fat Greek yoghurt.
- ¼ tsp Dijon mustard.
- 1 tsp chopped chives.
- 1 tsp lemon juice (fresh lemon wedge or bottled lemon juice).

Serve with:
- 1 round tomato.
- Sea salt and black pepper.
- 100g ham, sliced.
- 100g spinach.
- Vegetables of choice - see transformation food tables.

METHOD

1. Slice the tomato in half and season with sea salt and black pepper. Place on a grill pan and grill for 5 minutes under a high heat.

2. Start to poach the eggs following the *'Basic Poached Eggs'* method.

3. While the eggs cook, start to prepare the sauce. Place a small saucepan over a low heat and add the Greek yoghurt, Dijon mustard and chopped chives. Mix together and adjust the heat so that the sauce gently simmers.

4. When the eggs are ready, add the lemon juice to the sauce and then remove the pan from the heat.

5. Lay the spinach on your plate and top with the tomatoes, ham and poached eggs. Pour over the sauce and serve with any extra vegetables of your choice.

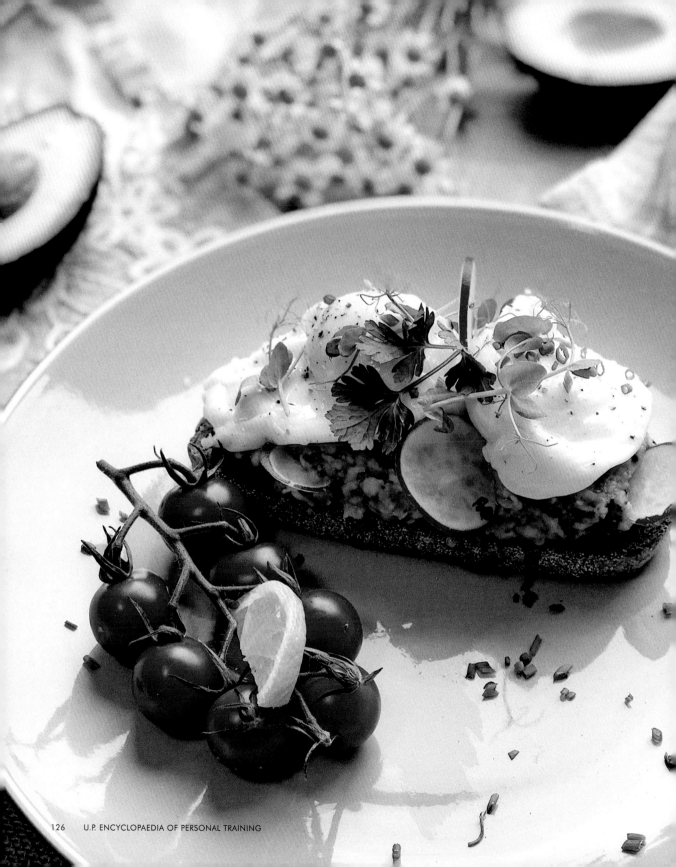

BREAKFASTS

POACHED EGGS WITH SOURDOUGH AND AVOCADO

PREP TIME: Under 10 mins.
COOK TIME: Under 10 mins.

CALORIES	PROTEIN	FAT	CARBS
380 kCal	20 g	20 g	30 g

EQUIPMENT

- Digital food scales.
- Large non-stick saucepan with a lid.
- Slotted spoon.
- Toaster or grill.
- Steamer or boil vegetables in saucepan.
- Mixing bowl.

INGREDIENTS

- 2 medium whole eggs.
- 1 tsp white wine vinegar.

Serve with:

- 1 slice sourdough toast.
- ½ avocado, peeled.
- ½ tsp chilli flakes.
- Sea salt and black pepper.
- 100g spinach.
- Vegetables of choice - see transformation food tables.

METHOD

1. Start to poach the eggs following the *'Basic Poached Eggs'* method.

2. While the eggs cook, toast or grill the sourdough and steam the spinach until tender.

3. Add the avocado to a mixing bowl. Season with sea salt, black pepper and chilli flakes.

4. Spread the avocado onto the toasted sourdough and top with the poached eggs and steamed spinach. Serve along with any extra vegetables of your choice.

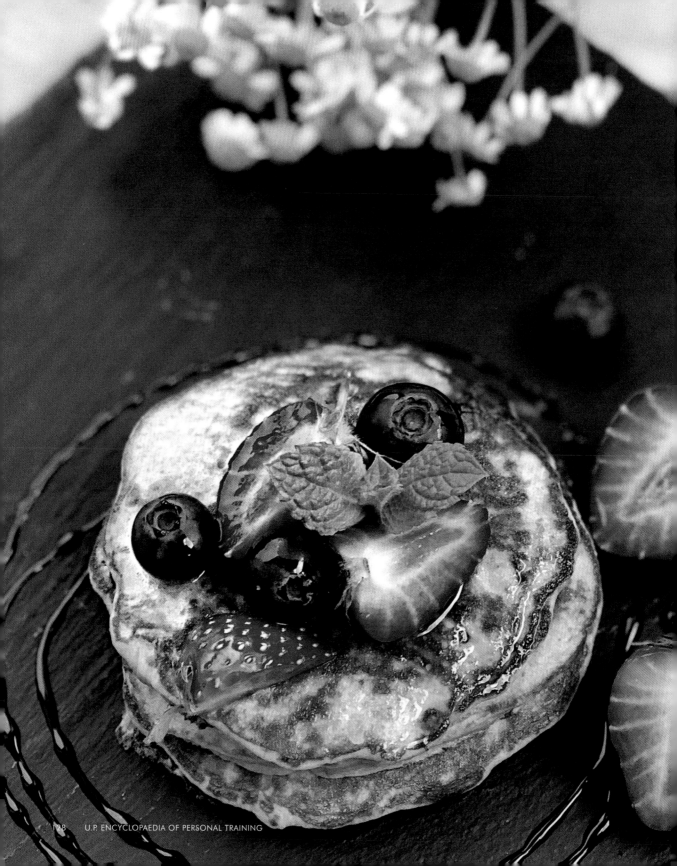

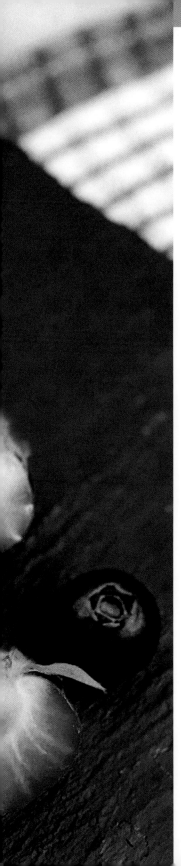

BREAKFASTS

HOW TO MAKE PANCAKES

PREP TIME: Under 10 mins.
COOK TIME: Under 10 mins.

CALORIES	PROTEIN	FAT	CARBS
245 kCal	35 g	5 g	15 g

EQUIPMENT

- Digital food scales.
- Blender or mixing bowl and whisk/fork.
- Large non-stick frying pan.
- Spatula.
- Ladle.

INGREDIENTS

Note: Makes 4 pancakes.

- 1 medium whole egg.
- 1 egg white or 2 tbsp liquid egg white.
- 1 banana, peeled.
- 25g whey protein (flavour of choice).
- 50ml almond milk.

METHOD

1. Combine all the ingredients in a blender or mixing bowl and beat until there are no lumps in the mixture.

2. Place a frying pan over medium-high heat. To test if the pan is ready, add ½teaspoon of pancake mix onto the centre. If the mixture bubbles around the edges, the pan is ready. If it bubbles vigorously and smokes a little, turn the heat down and retest after 30 seconds.

3. When the pan is ready, use the ladle to guide the mixture into the pan (make 1 pancake at a time if you only have a small pan).

4. When the edges begin to bubble, slide the spatula underneath the pancake and flip it over onto the other side.

5. Leave the pancake for 30 seconds and then use your spatula to remove from the pan.

6. Repeat steps 3-6 until you have used up all the pancake mix.

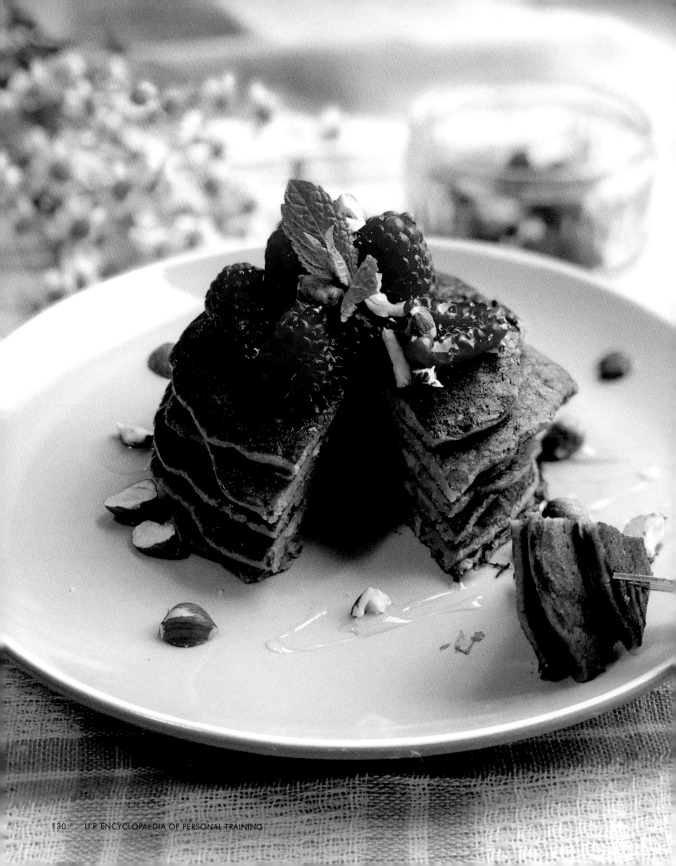

BREAKFASTS

U.P. CHOCOTRIENTS PANCAKES

PREP TIME: Under 10 mins.
COOK TIME: Under 10 mins.

CALORIES	PROTEIN	FAT	CARBS
355 kCal	40 g	15 g	15 g

EQUIPMENT

- Digital food scales.
- Blender or mixing bowl and whisk/fork.
- Large non-stick frying pan.
- Spatula.
- Ladle.
- Mixing bowl.

INGREDIENTS

- 1 medium whole egg.
- 1 egg white or 2 tbsp liquid egg white.
- 1 banana, peeled.
- 25g chocolate whey protein.
- 50ml almond milk.
- ½ scoop U.P. Chocotrients.

For the sauce:
- 1 tsp coconut oil, melted.
- ½ scoop U.P. Chocotrients.

Serve with:
- 1 tsp chopped hazelnuts.
- Fruit, nuts and seeds of choice - see transformation food tables.

METHOD

1. Follow the *'Basic Pancake'* method to prepare the pancakes using all the ingredients listed.

2. To prepare the chocolate sauce, combine the U.P. Chocotrients with the coconut oil in a mixing bowl and stir well.

3. Pour the sauce over the pancakes. Top with chopped hazelnuts and serve with any extra fruit, nuts or seeds of your choice.

Note:
U.P. Chocotrients is available on our website, www.upfitness.com/shop

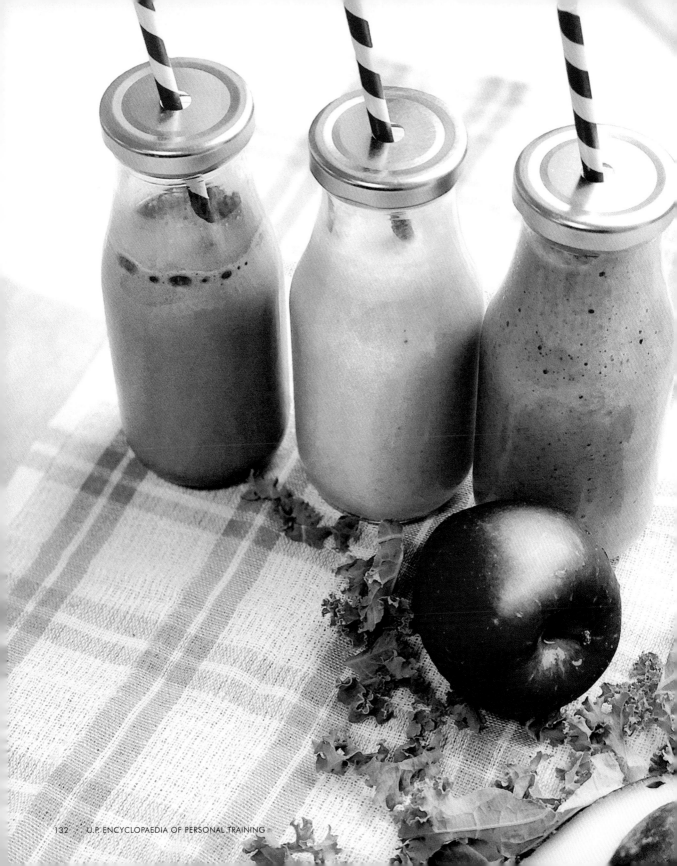

BREAKFASTS

PROTEIN SHAKES

PEANUT BUTTER BANANA

CALORIES	PROTEIN	FAT	CARBS
270 kCal	30 g	10 g	15 g

INGREDIENTS

- 35g vanilla whey protein.
- 1 banana, peeled.
- 10g smooth peanut butter.
- 100ml almond milk.
- 100ml water.
- Optional: ice cubes.

SUPER GREEN SMOOTHIE

CALORIES	PROTEIN	FAT	CARBS
160 kCal	30 g	0 g	10 g

INGREDIENTS

- 35g vanilla whey protein.
- 50g spinach.
- 50g kale.
- 50g pear.
- 1 tsp chopped fresh mint.
- ½ tsp ground root ginger.
- 200ml water.
- Optional: ice cubes.

NUTELLA

CALORIES	PROTEIN	FAT	CARBS
230 kCal	30 g	10 g	5 g

INGREDIENTS

- 35g chocolate whey protein.
- 1 tsp hazelnut butter or 15g hazelnuts.
- 100ml almond milk.
- 100ml water.
- Optional: ice cubes.

EQUIPMENT

- Digital food scales.
- Blender.

METHOD

1. Add all the ingredients into a blender and pulse until smooth.
2. Enjoy.

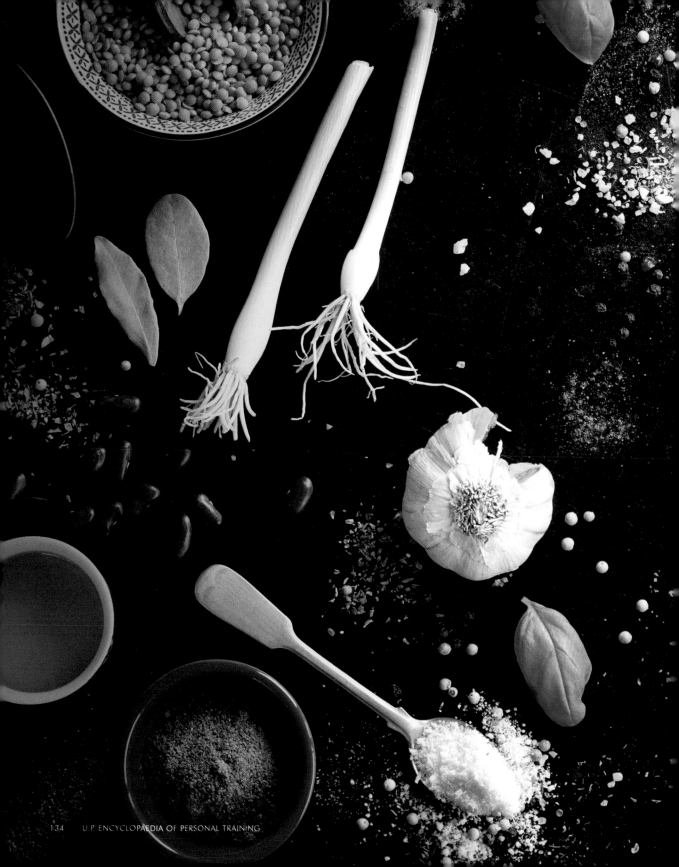

LOW-CARB MAIN MEALS

Chinese Prawn Stir-fry

Mexican Venison Chilli
and Smashed Avocado

Teriyaki Salmon

Steak and Chimichurri

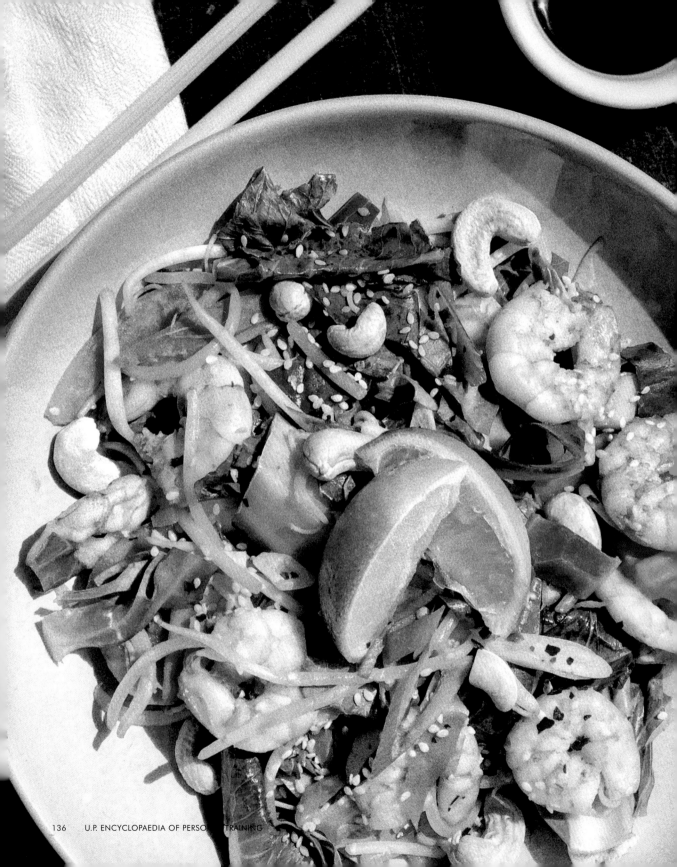

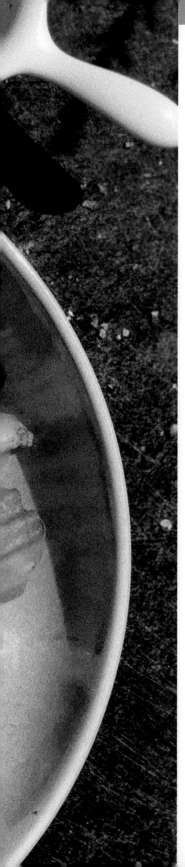

LOW-CARB MAIN MEALS

CHINESE PRAWN STIR-FRY

PREP TIME: 1 hour (marinade).
COOK TIME: Under 10 mins.

CALORIES	PROTEIN	FAT	CARBS
270 kCal	35 g	10 g	10 g

EQUIPMENT

- Digital food scales.
- Wok or large non-stick frying pan.
- Spatula.
- Mixing bowl.

INGREDIENTS

- Low-calorie cooking spray.
- 150g raw king prawns.
- 50g carrot, sliced.
- 50g bean sprouts.
- 1 spring onion, sliced.
- 10g cashews, crushed.

For the marinade:
- 1 tbsp dark soy sauce.
- 1 tsp honey.
- 1 tsp rice vinegar.
- 1 tsp lime juice (fresh lime wedge or bottled lime juice).
- ½ red chilli, deseeded.

Serve with:
- Vegetables of choice - see transformation food tables.

METHOD

1. To prepare the marinade, combine the soy sauce, honey, rice vinegar, lime juice and red chilli in a mixing bowl.

2. Marinate the king prawns in the mixture for a minimum of 1 hour in the fridge.

3. Place a wok or frying pan lightly coated with low-calorie cooking spray over high heat. Add the king prawns and stir-fry for 5 minutes.

4. Add the carrot and beansprouts and stir-fry until the prawns are cooked through.

5. Remove the pan from the heat and serve topped with sliced spring onion, crushed cashews and vegetables of your choice.

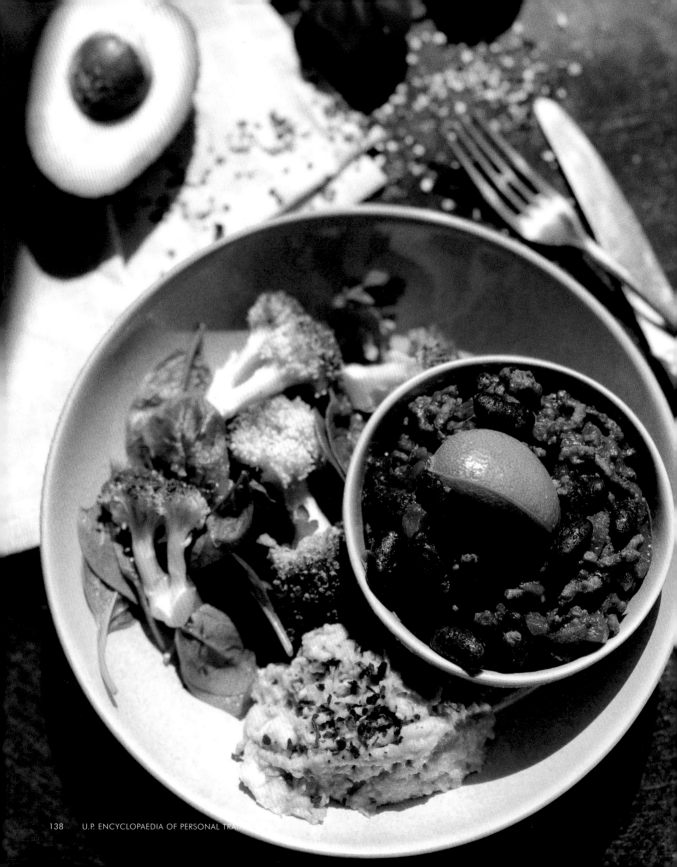

LOW-CARB MAIN MEALS

MEXICAN VENISON CHILLI AND SMASHED AVOCADO

	CALORIES	PROTEIN	FAT	CARBS
PREP TIME: Under 10 mins. **COOK TIME:** Under 30 mins.	375 kCal	40 g	15 g	20 g

EQUIPMENT

- Digital food scales.
- Large non-stick saucepan.
- Steamer or boil vegetables in saucepan.
- Mixing bowl.

INGREDIENTS

- Low-calorie cooking spray.
- ½ large onion, diced.
- 2 garlic cloves, minced or 2 tsp garlic paste.
- 1 red chilli, deseeded.
- 1 round tomato, quartered.
- 1 tsp smoked paprika.
- 1 tsp cumin.
- 150g minced venison.
- Sea salt and black pepper.
- ½ tsp instant coffee granules.
- 100g tomato passata.
- 1 tsp balsamic vinegar.
- 60g drained kidney beans.

Serve with:
- ½ avocado, peeled.
- 1 tsp chopped fresh parsley.
- 1 tsp lime juice (fresh lime wedge or bottled lime juice.
- 50g spinach.
- 50g broccoli.
- Vegetables of choice - see transformation food tables.

METHOD

1. Place a saucepan lightly coated with low-calorie cooking spray over medium-high heat. Add the onion, garlic, chilli, tomato, smoked paprika and cumin. Combine well and sauté for 5 minutes.

2. Add the minced venison and stir-fry until cooked through.

3. Add the instant coffee and combine well.

4. Add the tomato passata and balsamic vinegar and leave to simmer on low heat for 10 minutes uncovered.

5. As the sauce reduces and thickens, add the kidney beans and cook for a further 5 minutes.

6. While the chilli cooks, mash the avocado in a mixing bowl and combine with the fresh parsley and lime juice. Season with sea salt and black pepper.

7. Steam the broccoli until tender and add to your plate on a bed of spinach.

8. Remove the saucepan from the heat and serve the chilli on top of the vegetables. Top with the mashed avocado and add any extra vegetables of your choice.

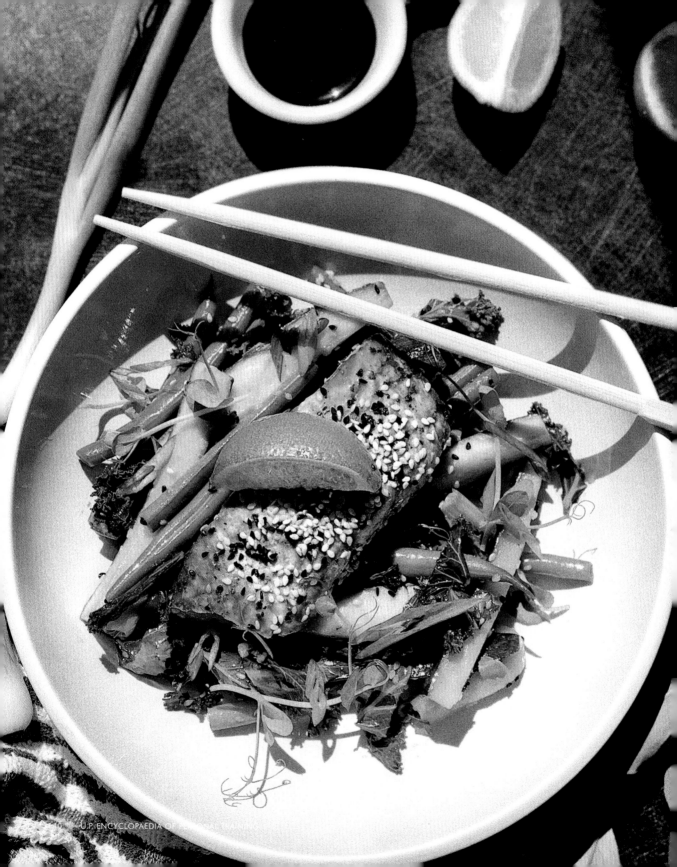

LOW-CARB MAIN MEALS

TERIYAKI SALMON

PREP TIME: 1 hour (marinade).
COOK TIME: Under 30 mins.

CALORIES	PROTEIN	FAT	CARBS
365 kCal	30 g	25 g	5 g

EQUIPMENT

- Digital food scales.
- Mixing bowl.
- Large non-stick saucepan.
- Baking tray.
- Tin foil.
- Steamer or boil vegetables in saucepan.

INGREDIENTS

- 1 salmon fillet (roughly 150g).
- 1 tsp onion seeds.

For the marinade:
- 1 tsp dark soy sauce.
- 1 tsp ginger paste.
- 1 tsp garlic paste.
- ½ tsp honey.
- 1 tsp sesame oil.

Serve with:
- 50g courgette.
- 50g green beans.
- 50g kale.
- 1 tsp sesame seeds.
- 1 lime wedge.
- Vegetables of choice - see transformation food tables.

METHOD

1. To prepare the marinade, combine the soy sauce, ginger paste, garlic paste, honey and sesame oil in a mixing bowl.

2. Marinate the salmon in the mixture for a minimum of 1 hour in the fridge.

3. Preheat your oven to 160°C (fan 140°C/gas mark 3).

4. Lay the marinated salmon on a foil-lined baking tray, top with onion seeds and cover with foil.

5. Roast the salmon in the oven until cooked through to your liking in the centre.

6. Steam the courgette, green beans and kale until tender. Then, sprinkle over the sesame seeds and roast on a baking tray in the oven for 5 minutes.

7. Serve the salmon alongside the vegetables. Add a lime wedge to garnish and any extra vegetables of your choice.

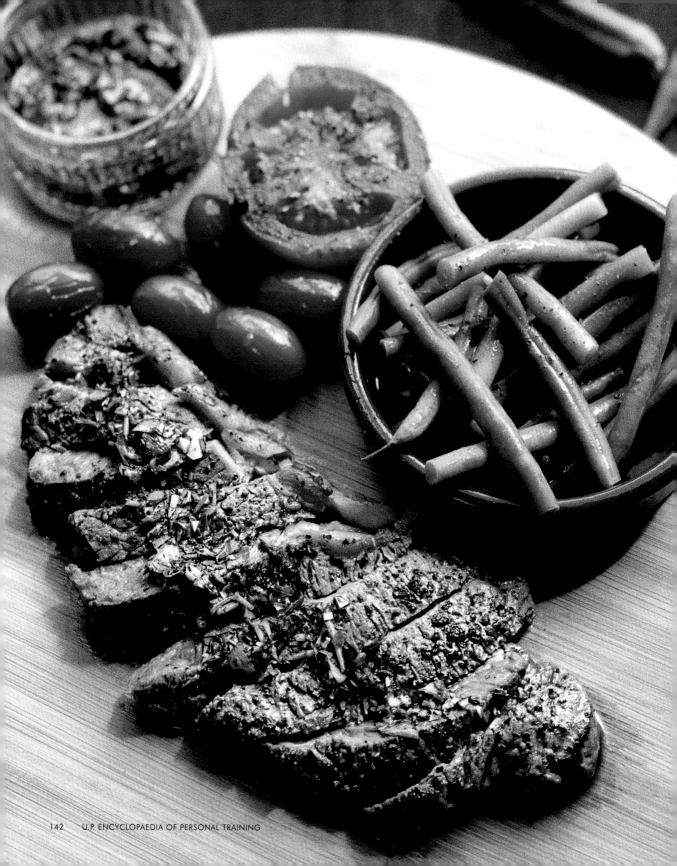

STEAK AND CHIMICHURRI

EQUIPMENT

- Digital food scales.
- Griddle pan or large non-stick frying pan.
- Steamer or boil vegetables in saucepan.
- Blender or food processor.
- Mixing bowl.

INGREDIENTS

- Low-calorie cooking spray.
- 1 sirloin steak (roughly 150g).

For the marinade:
- 1 garlic clove, minced or 1 tsp garlic paste.
- 1 tsp lemon juice (fresh lemon wedge or bottled lemon juice).
- 1 tsp olive oil.
- ½ tsp chilli flakes.
- Sea salt and black pepper.

For the chimichurri (makes 2 portions):
- 25g chopped fresh parsley.
- 1 garlic clove, minced or 1 tsp garlic paste.
- ½ tsp dried oregano.
- 50ml olive oil.
- 1 tbsp lemon juice.
- 1 tsp white wine vinegar.
- 1 tbsp honey.

Serve with:
- 50g tomatoes.
- 50g spinach.
- Vegetables of choice - see transformation food tables.

PREP TIME: 1 hour (marinade).
COOK TIME: Under 10 mins.

CALORIES	PROTEIN	FAT	CARBS
470 kCal	40 g	30 g	10 g

Note: Based on 1 serving of chimichurri.

METHOD

1. To prepare the marinade, combine the garlic, lemon juice, olive oil and chilli flakes in a mixing bowl. Season with sea salt and black pepper.

2. Marinate the steak in the mixture for a minimum of 1 hour in the fridge.

3. To prepare the chimichurri, combine all the ingredients in a food processor and pulse until the mixture is smooth and vibrant green.

4. 10 minutes before serving, remove the steak from the fridge and heat a griddle pan or frying pan lightly coated with low-calorie cooking spray over high heat.

5. Sear the steak for 1-2 minutes on each side depending on how well-done you like your steak (resist the urge to constantly flip the steak while cooking!). Then, leave to rest on a chopping board for 5 minutes.

6. While the steak rests, steam the spinach until tender.

7. Serve the steak topped with the chimichurri and a side of vegetables.

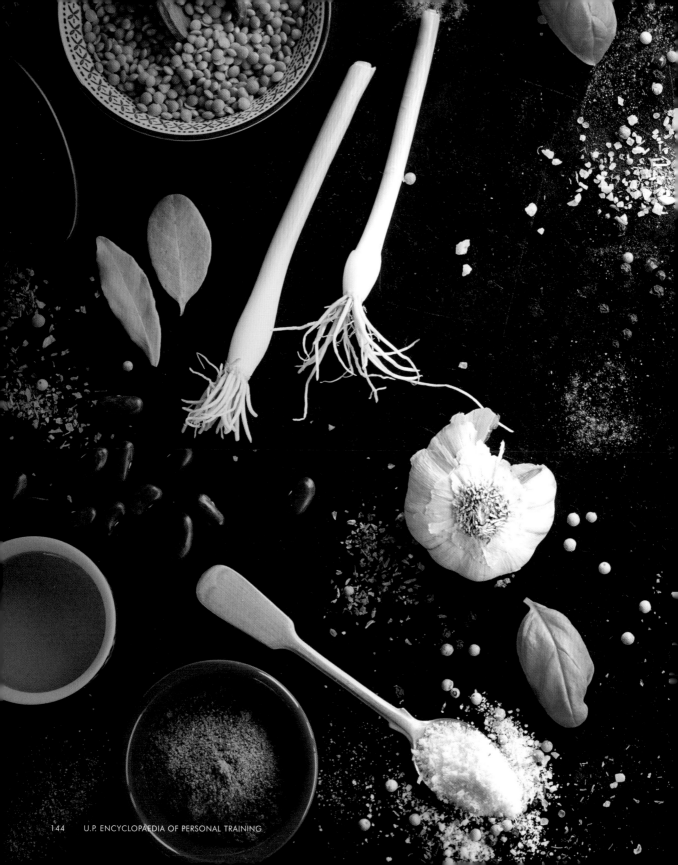

HIGH-CARB MAIN MEALS

Chicken Fried Rice

Haddock and Sweet Potato Chips

Beef Burgers and Sweet
Potato Wedges

Beef Ragu and Wholegrain Spaghetti

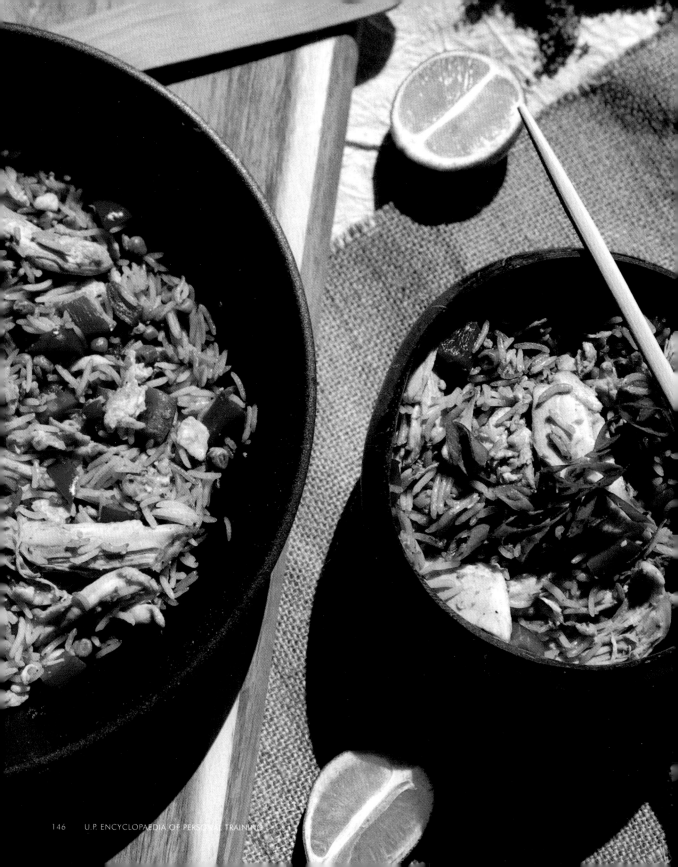

HIGH-CARB MAIN MEALS

CHICKEN FRIED RICE

PREP TIME: Under 10 mins.
COOK TIME: Under 30 mins.

CALORIES	PROTEIN	FAT	CARBS
435 kCal	45 g	15 g	30 g

EQUIPMENT

- Digital food scales.
- Whisk or fork.
- Baking tray.
- Wok or large non-stick frying pan.

INGREDIENTS

- 1 chicken breast (roughly 150g).
- 1 tsp dark soy sauce.
- 1 tsp olive oil.
- 125g cooked basmati rice (uncooked weight: roughly 25g).
- 50g peppers (any colour), diced.
- 1 medium whole egg, whisked.
- 1 spring onion, sliced.
- 50g kale.
- 50g broccoli.

Serve with:

- Vegetables of choice - see transformation food tables.

METHOD

1. Preheat your oven to 200°C (fan 180°C/gas mark 6).

2. Roast the chicken breast on a baking tray in the oven until it is cooked through.

3. Remove the cooked chicken from the oven and allow to cool. Next, use 2 forks (or your fingers) to tear the chicken into thin strips.

4. Place a wok or frying pan over medium-high heat. Add the soy sauce and olive oil and tilt the pan to get an even coating.

5. Add the cooked rice, chicken, pepper, kale and broccoli to the pan. Cook for 5 minutes stirring occasionally.

6. Push all the ingredients to one side of the pan and add the whisked egg. Scramble the egg and then combine with the rest of the ingredients.

7. Remove the pan from the heat and serve topped with sliced spring onion and any extra vegetables of your choice.

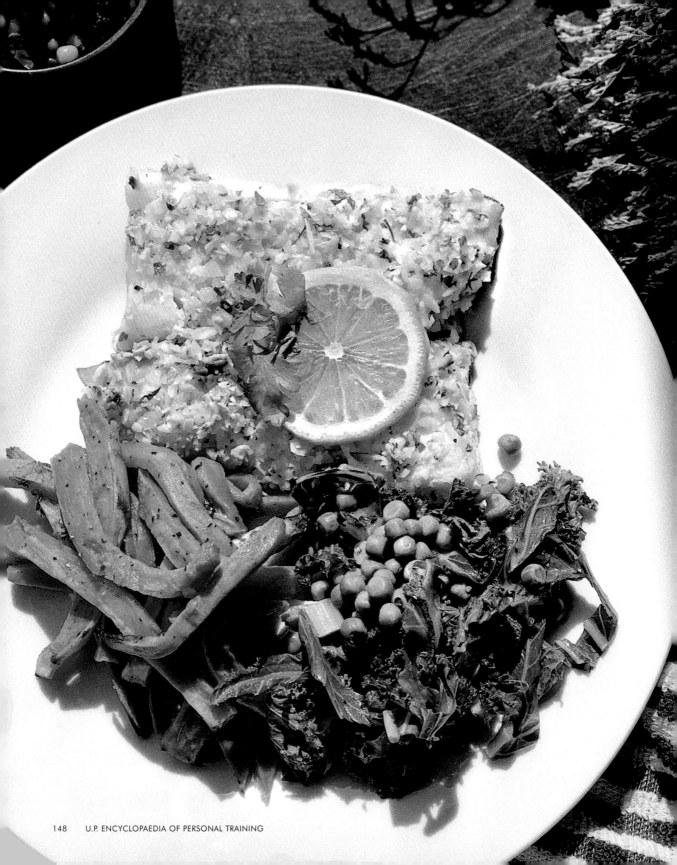

HIGH-CARB MAIN MEALS

HADDOCK AND SWEET POTATO CHIPS

PREP TIME: Under 10 mins.
COOK TIME: Under 30 mins.

CALORIES	PROTEIN	FAT	CARBS
435 kCal	40 g	15 g	35 g

EQUIPMENT

- Digital food scales.
- Blender or food processor.
- Steamer or boil vegetables in saucepan.
- Baking tray.
- Regular non-stick saucepan.

INGREDIENTS

- 15g flaked almonds.
- 1 tsp chopped fresh parsley.
- Sea salt and black pepper.
- 1 haddock fillet (roughly 200g).
- 1 tsp lemon juice (fresh lemon wedge or bottled lemon juice).
- 150g sweet potato.

Serve with:
- 50g petit pois peas.
- 50g green beans.
- 50g kale.
- 1 tsp chopped fresh mint.
- 1 tsp butter.
- 1 lemon wedge.
- Vegetables of choice - see transformation food tables.

METHOD

1. Preheat your oven to 160°C (fan 140°C/gas mark 3).

2. Add the flaked almonds to a blender or food processor and blend until they are coarse but not the consistency of ground almonds.

3. Add the parsley, season with sea salt and black pepper and blend for an extra 5-10 seconds to create an almond 'crumb'.

4. Drizzle the lemon juice evenly over the haddock fillet and then lay the fillet in the almond crumb on both sides to coat.

5. Slice the sweet potato lengthways to create chips and season with sea salt and black pepper.

6. Roast the sweet potato chips and haddock together on a baking tray in the oven for 20 minutes.

7. Boil the petit pois peas and steam the green beans and kale until tender.

8. Mix the vegetables in the saucepan along with the fresh mint and butter.

9. Serve with a wedge of lemon to garnish and any extra vegetables of your choice.

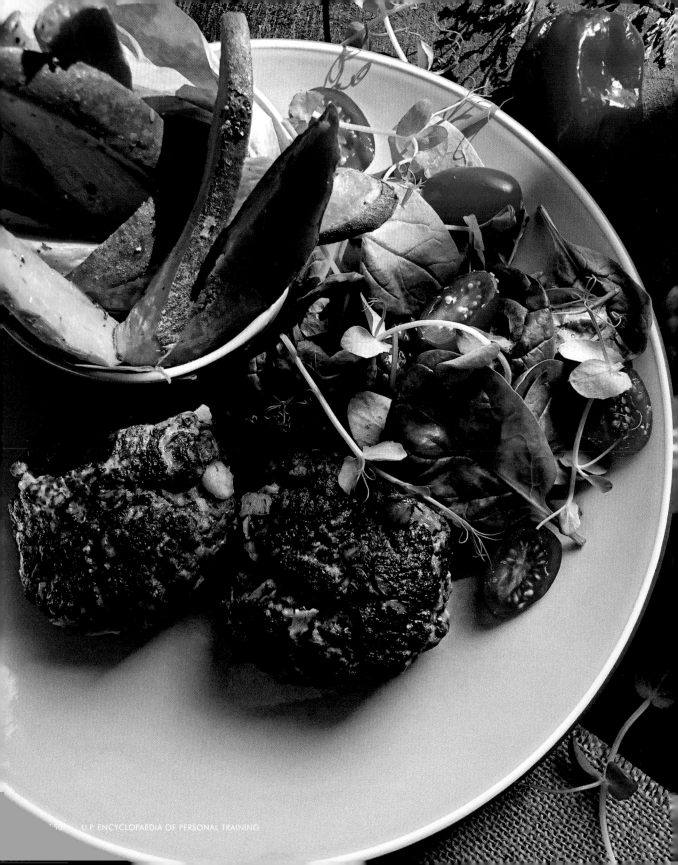

HIGH-CARB MAIN MEALS

BEEF BURGERS AND SWEET POTATO WEDGES

PREP TIME: Under 10 mins.
COOK TIME: Under 30 mins.

	CALORIES	PROTEIN	FAT	CARBS
	455 kCal	45 g	15 g	35 g

EQUIPMENT

- Digital food scales.
- Whisk or fork.
- Large non-stick frying pan.
- Baking tray.
- 2 Large mixing bowls.

INGREDIENTS

- 150g lean minced beef (10% fat).
- 1 medium whole egg, whisked.
- 1 tsp garlic granules.
- 1 tsp onion granules.
- 1 tsp smoked paprika.
- 1 tsp wholegrain mustard.
- 1 tsp chopped fresh parsley.
- Sea salt and black pepper.
- Low-calorie cooking spray.
- 150g sweet potato.
- 1 tsp chopped chives.

Serve with:
- 50g spinach.
- 50g watercress.
- 50g tomatoes.
- Vegetables of choice - see transformation food tables.

METHOD

1. Preheat your oven to 180°C (fan 160°C/gas mark 4).

2. Add the minced beef, whisked egg, garlic granules, onion granules, smoked paprika and mustard to a large mixing bowl and combine thoroughly.

3. Sprinkle the chopped parsley over the mixture and season with sea salt and black pepper.

4. With slightly damp hands, shape the mixture into 2 equal sized patties.

5. Place a frying pan lightly coated with low-calorie cooking spray over high heat and sear the burgers for 2 minutes on each side.

6. Roast the burgers on a baking tray in the oven for 10-15 minutes (depending on how well-done you like your burgers).

7. Slice the sweet potato lengthways into wedges and season with chopped chives, sea salt and black pepper.

8. Roast the wedges on a baking tray in the oven for 20 minutes.

9. While the burgers and wedges roast, combine the spinach, watercress and tomatoes in a clean mixing bowl.

10. Serve everything together with any extra vegetables of your choice.

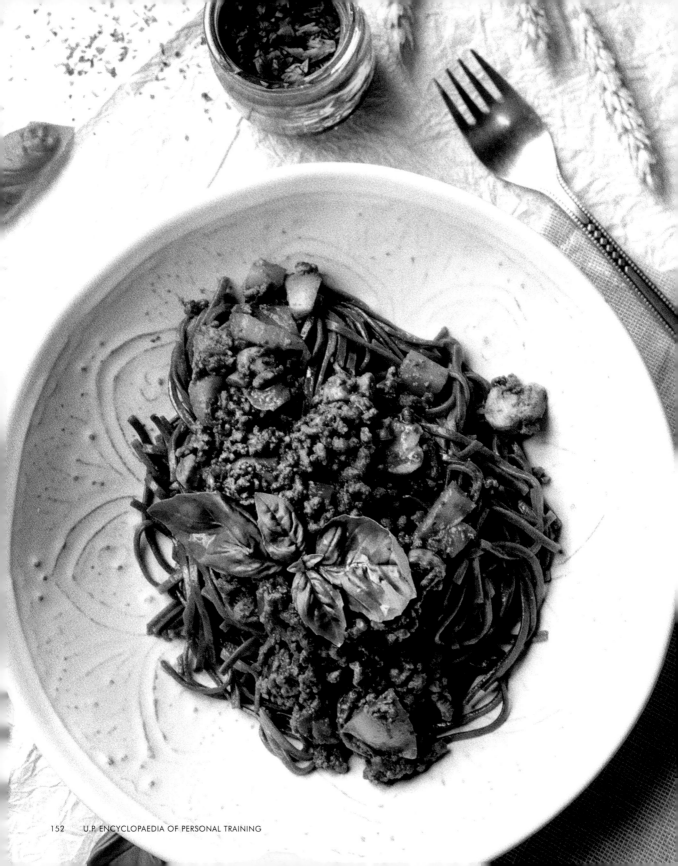

HIGH-CARB MAIN MEALS

BEEF RAGU AND WHOLEGRAIN SPAGHETTI

PREP TIME: Under 10 mins.
COOK TIME: 30 mins – 1 hour.

CALORIES	PROTEIN	FAT	CARBS
475 kCal	45 g	15 g	40 g

EQUIPMENT

- Digital food scales.
- Large non-stick frying pan.
- Regular non-stick saucepan.

INGREDIENTS

- Low-calorie cooking spray.
- 1 garlic clove, minced or 1 tsp garlic paste.
- ¼ white onion, diced.
- 1 tsp dried oregano.
- 1 tsp smoked paprika.
- 1 tsp balsamic vinegar.
- 150g lean minced beef (10% fat).
- 50g peppers (any colour), diced.
- 50g mushrooms, sliced.
- 100g chopped tomatoes.
- 50g wholegrain spaghetti.
- 1 tsp shredded basil.

Serve with:

- Vegetables of choice - see transformation food tables.

METHOD

1. Place a frying pan lightly coated with low-calorie cooking spray over medium-high heat. Add the garlic and onion and sauté for 1-2 minutes.

2. Add the oregano, paprika and balsamic vinegar and combine well.

3. Add the minced beef and stir-fry until cooked through.

4. Add the peppers and mushrooms and stir-fry for up to 5 minutes until tender.

5. Pour over the chopped tomatoes, stir well and leave to simmer on low heat for 20 minutes uncovered.

6. While the ragu reduces, bring a pan of water to the boil and cook the spaghetti as instructed on the packaging.

7. Drain off the spaghetti, add to your plate and season with sea salt and black pepper.

8. Sprinkle the basil over the ragu (which should be a thick but saucy consistency) and toss through.

9. Remove the pan from the heat and serve the ragu on top of the spaghetti along with any vegetables of your choice.

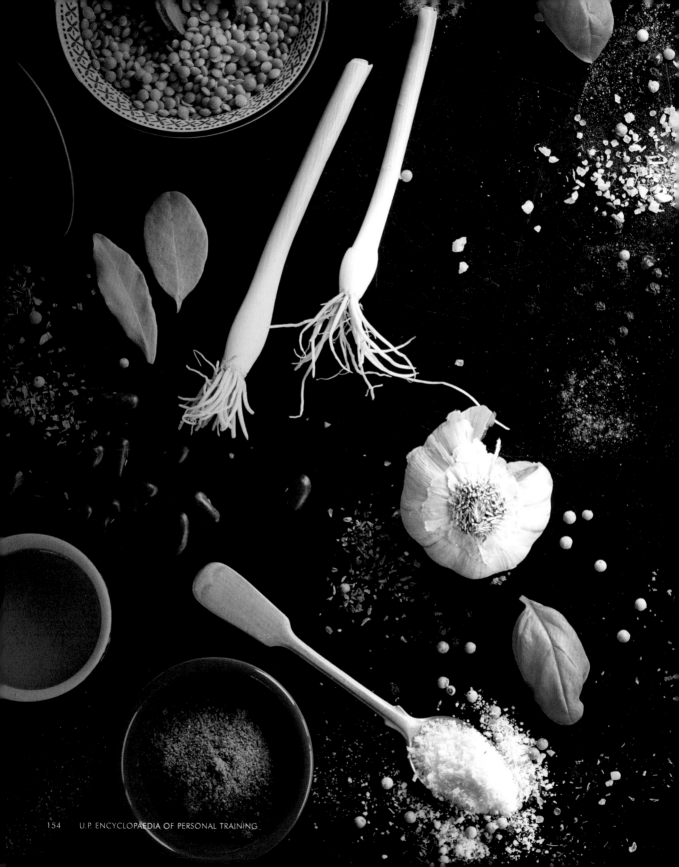

VEGETABLES AND SALADS

Roasted Mediterranean Vegetables

Cauliflower Rice

Spiralized Sesame Noodles

Salads and Dressings

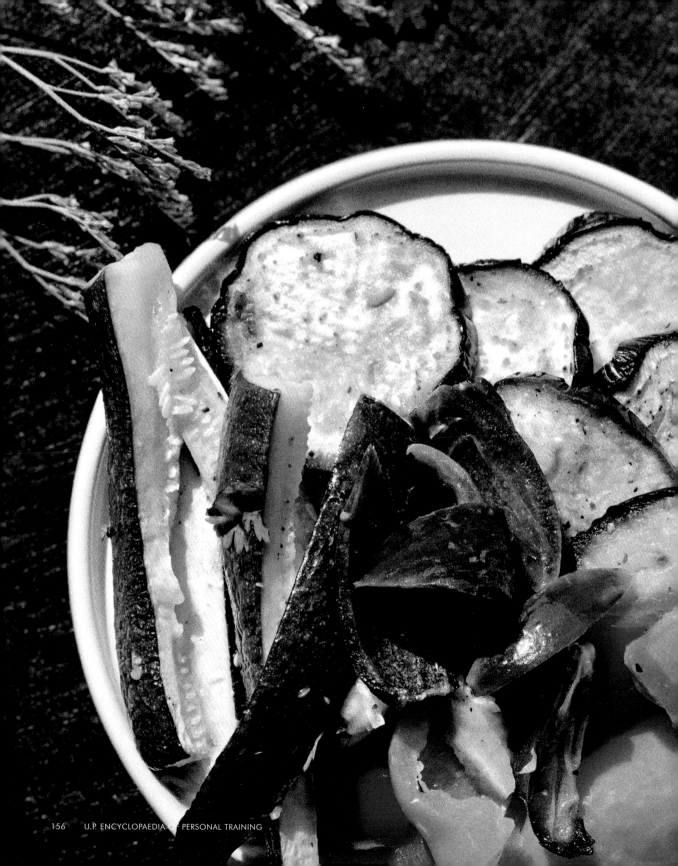

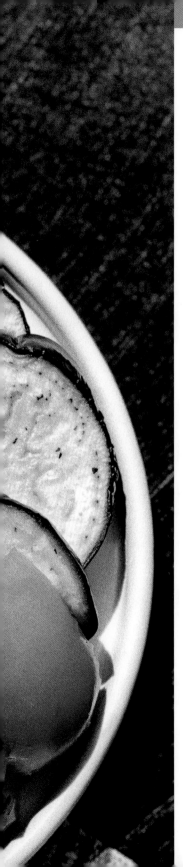

VEGETABLES AND SALADS

ROASTED MEDITERRANEAN VEGETABLES

	CALORIES	PROTEIN	FAT	CARBS
PREP TIME: Under 10 mins. **COOK TIME:** Under 30 mins.	60 kCal	5 g	0 g	10 g

EQUIPMENT

- Baking tray.

INGREDIENTS

- 100g aubergine, diced (large chunks).
- 100g courgette, diced (large chunks).
- 100g peppers, diced (large chunks).
- ½ red onion, diced (large chunks).
- Low-calorie cooking spray.
- ½ tsp smoked paprika.
- ½ tsp dried basil.
- Sea salt and black pepper.
- 1 tsp red wine vinegar.

METHOD

1. Preheat your oven to 180°C (fan 160°C/gas mark 4).

2. Add the aubergine, courgette, peppers and red onion to a baking tray.

3. Lightly coat the vegetables with low-calorie cooking spray and season with smoked paprika, dried basil, sea salt and black pepper.

4. Roast the vegetables in the oven for 20 minutes.

5. Drizzle the red wine vinegar over the vegetables making sure they are evenly coated.

6. Roast the vegetables for an additional 5 minutes and serve as part of a recipe of your choice.

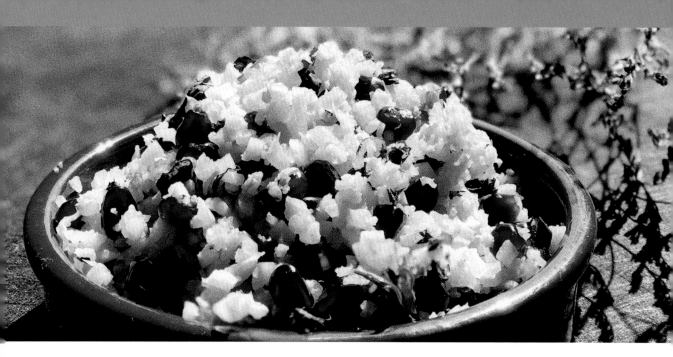

CAULIFLOWER RICE

PREP TIME: Under 10 mins.
COOK TIME: Under 10 mins.

CALORIES	PROTEIN	FAT	CARBS
60 kCal	5 g	0 g	10 g

EQUIPMENT

- Blender or food processor.
- Cling film

INGREDIENTS

- 150g cauliflower, chopped (florets).
- 1 tsp chopped fresh parsley.
- Sea salt and black pepper.
- 1 tsp pomegranate seeds.

METHOD

1. Add the cauliflower to a blender or food processor and pulse until it has a couscous-like consistency.

2. Season with fresh parsley, sea salt and black pepper.

3. Steam the cauliflower rice for 5 minutes. Alternatively, place in a bowl covered with cling film and microwave on full power for 5 minutes. Make sure to pierce holes in the cling film to allow hot air to escape.

4. Top with pomegranate seeds and serve in place of rice or couscous in a recipe of your choice.

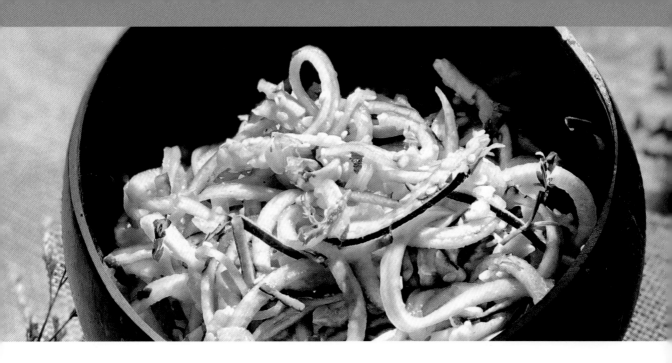

SPIRALIZED SESAME NOODLES

PREP TIME: Under 10 mins.
COOK TIME: Under 10 mins.

CALORIES	PROTEIN	FAT	CARBS
85 kCal	5 g	5 g	5 g

EQUIPMENT

- Spiralizer.
- Large non-stick frying pan.

INGREDIENTS

- 150g courgette.
- 1 tsp sesame oil.
- 1 tsp sesame seeds.
- Sea salt and black pepper.

METHOD

1. Feed the courgette through the spiralizer to create courgette noodles.

2. Place a frying pan over medium-high heat. Add the sesame oil and noodles and stir-fry for 3-4 minutes.

3. Sprinkle over the sesame seeds and season with sea salt and black pepper.

4. Remove the pan from the heat and serve the noodles in place of standard noodles or spaghetti in a recipe of your choice.

SALADS & DRESSING

Salads are an easy way to add fruit and vegetables to your meal plan and are staple meals in our transformation clients' diets.

ADDED CARBS	6
ADDED FATS	5
ADDED PROTEIN	4
ADDED COLOUR	3
ADDED CRUNCH	2
SALAD BASE	1

POSITIVES

- Low-calorie and high in fibre which makes them very filling.

- An easy way to add variety to your meal plan (and use up leftovers) by swapping in different ingredients.

- Minimal preparation time and easy to make multiple servings in one go.

(Note: restaurant salads are not automatically low-calorie options. Always ask for the dressing to be served on the side).

There is an almost unlimited number of potential salad combinations to try. Use the following graphic to start making a variety of fresh salads - do not be afraid to experiment!

GUIDELINES:

▶ You can prepare a salad to have as a starter, side-dish or as the main meal itself.

▶ Each table row is an example salad combination, but you do not have to stick to these, and can mix and match any of the ingredients together.

▶ There are no exact required portion sizes for each component, and you can customise them to meet your nutrition targets for a given meal.

▶ To save time, you can buy pre-washed and shredded salad bases and add extra ingredients on top.

SALAD BASE	ADDED CRUNCH	ADDED COLOUR	ADDED PROTEIN	ADDED FATS	ADDED CARBS
Spinach	Cucumber, sliced	Tomatoes	Chicken breast strips	Olives	Wholewheat pitta bread, sliced
Rocket	Peppers, sliced	Grated carrot	Tofu, diced	Toasted seeds	Quinoa
Kale	Radish, sliced	Beetroot	Steak strips	Feta, crumbled	Roasted butternut squash, diced
Watercress	Pear, sliced	Red onion	Boiled eggs, halved	Blue cheese, crumbled	Steamed sweet potato, diced
Mixed leaves	Green beans	Grilled aubergine	Tuna chunks	Walnuts, crushed	Chickpeas

Once you have made your salad, the next step is to add a dressing. You can use store-bought dressings or single-ingredient options like olive oil and lemon juice.

Alternatively, you can try making a dressing from scratch. To make a simple salad dressing, all you need is an oil (e.g. olive oil), acid (e.g. balsamic vinegar) and a selection of herbs (e.g. parsley) and sweet ingredients (e.g. honey) for added flavour. For a quick and easy method, select one ingredient from each column in the table below, add everything to a mixing bowl and whisk with a fork for 30 seconds to combine.

BASE (2-3 TBSP)	Added Acid (1 tsp)	Added Herbs	Added Sweetness
Olive oil	Balsamic Vinegar	Parsley	Honey
Rapeseed oil	Dijon mustard	Chives	Orange juice
Avocado oil	Lemon juice	Basil	-
-	-	Thyme	-

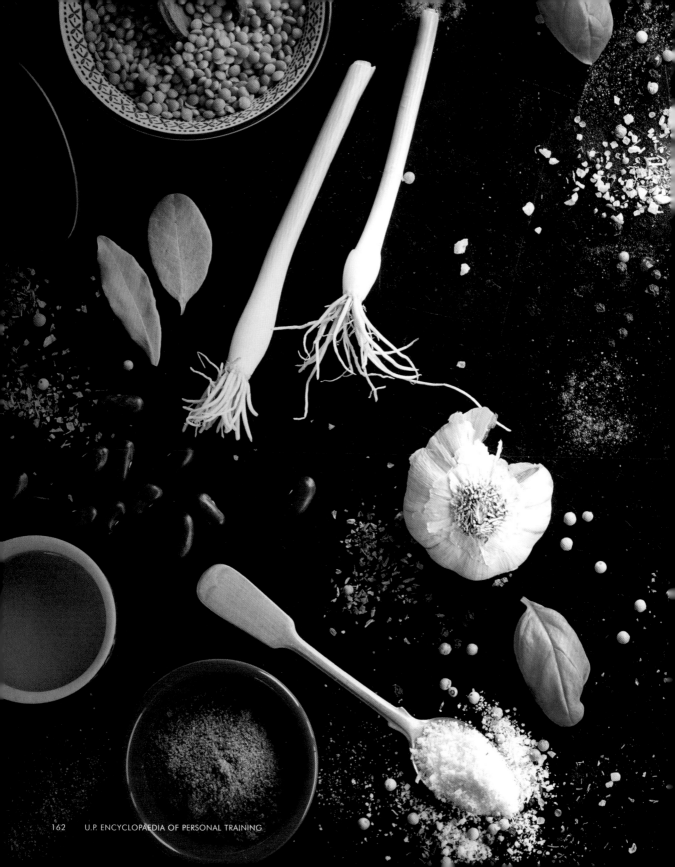

REFEED INSPIRATION

Burrito

Pizza

Chocolate 'Ice Cream'

Avocado Chocolate Mousse

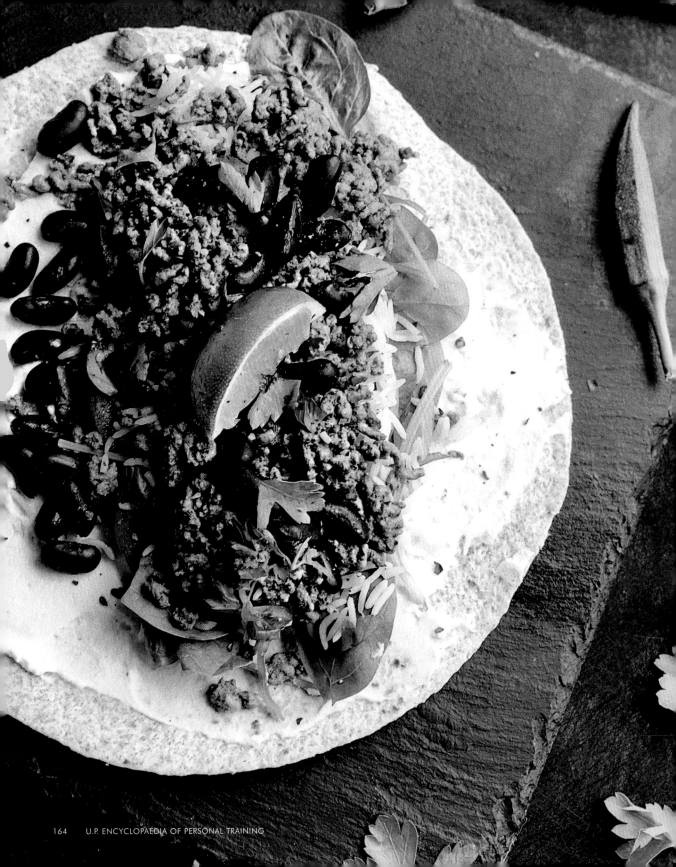

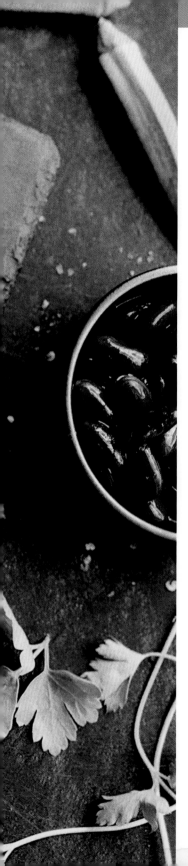

BURRITO

PREP TIME: Under 10 mins.
COOK TIME: Under 30 mins.

CALORIES	PROTEIN	FAT	CARBS
580 kCal	50 g	20 g	50 g

EQUIPMENT

- Digital food scales.
- Large non-stick frying pan.

INGREDIENTS

- ½ garlic clove, minced or 1 tsp garlic paste.
- ½ tsp smoked paprika.
- 150g lean minced beef (10% fat).
- 1 tortilla wrap.
- 20g ricotta cheese.
- 50g spinach.
- 50g tomatoes, sliced.
- 100g cooked basmati rice (uncooked weight: roughly 20g).
- 50g drained black beans.

Serve with:

- Vegetables of choice – see transformation food tables.

METHOD

1. Place a frying pan over medium-high heat and add the garlic.

2. Add the minced beef and smoked paprika and stir-fry until cooked through.

3. While the minced beef cooks, lay out the tortilla wrap and spread the ricotta cheese evenly on top.

4. Add the spinach, tomatoes, cooked rice and black beans to the tortilla.

5. Top with the cooked beef and wrap into a burrito. Serve with a side of vegetables of your choice.

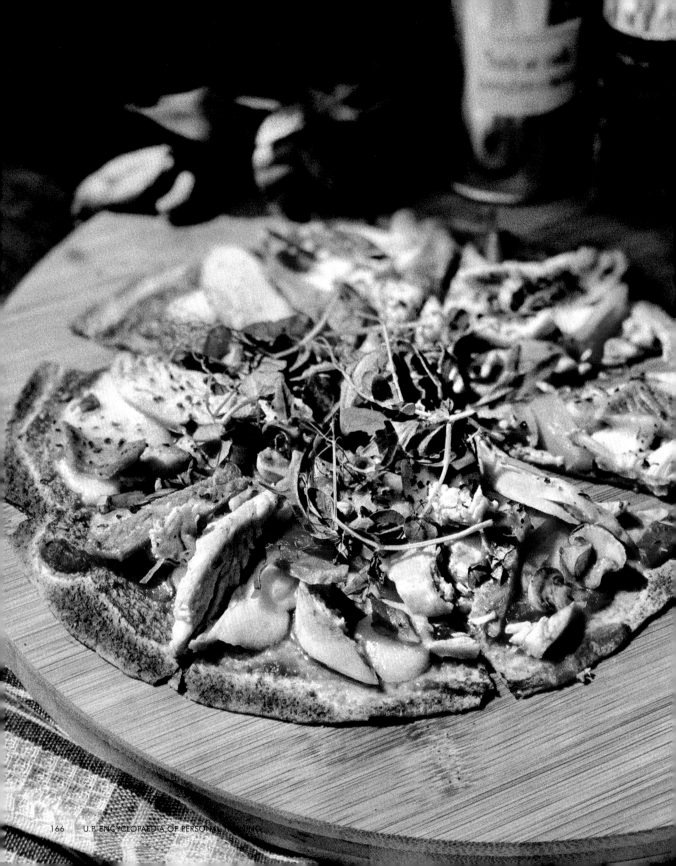

REFEED INSPIRATION

PIZZA

PREP TIME: Under 10 mins.
COOK TIME: Under 30 mins.

CALORIES	PROTEIN	FAT	CARBS
435 kCal	40 g	15 g	35 g

EQUIPMENT

- Digital food scales.
- Large non-stick frying pan.
- Baking tray.
- Grill pan.

INGREDIENTS

- 50g mushrooms, sliced
- 1 tortilla wrap.
- 50g tomato passata.
- 1 tsp dried basil.
- 100g chicken breast.
- 2 bacon slices.
- Low-calorie cooking spray.
- 50g peppers (any colour), diced.
- 25g mozzarella.
- 50g spinach.

Serve with:

- Vegetables of choice - see transformation food tables.

METHOD

1. Preheat your oven to 200°C (fan 180°C/gas mark 6).

2. Roast the chicken breast on a baking tray until cooked through.

3. Remove the cooked chicken from the oven and allow to cool. Then, use 2 forks (or your fingers) to tear the chicken into thin strips.

4. Prepare the bacon by grilling under a high heat until crispy, then slice into thin strips.

5. Place a frying pan lightly coated with low-calorie cooking spray over medium-high heat. Add the mushrooms and stir-fry for 2 minutes.

6. Lay out the tortilla wrap and spread the tomato passata evenly on top. Sprinkle over the dried basil and mushrooms.

7. Add the chicken, bacon, peppers and mozzarella to the tortilla.

8. Grill the tortilla under a high heat until the edges begin to brown.

9. Top with spinach and serve with vegetables of your choice.

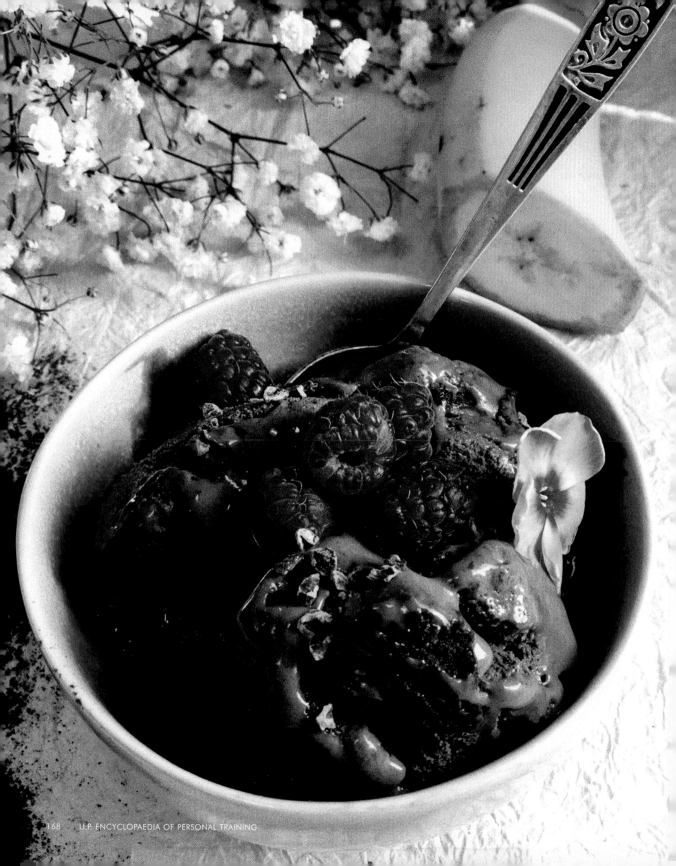

REFEED INSPIRATION

CHOCOLATE 'ICE CREAM'

PREP TIME: Under 10 mins.
COOL TIME: 1 - 2 hours.

CALORIES	PROTEIN	FAT	CARBS
100 kCal	10 g	2 g	10 g

EQUIPMENT

- Digital food scales.
- Spatula.
- Blender or food processor.
- Grater.
- Plastic container.

INGREDIENTS

Note: makes 4 portions.

- 1 frozen banana, peeled and sliced.
- 200g 0% fat Greek yoghurt.
- 25g chocolate whey protein.
- 1 tbsp unsweetened cocoa powder.
- 75ml skimmed milk.
- 10g 70-90% dark chocolate.

Serve with:

- Fruit, nuts and seeds of choice –
  see transformation food tables.

METHOD

1. Add the banana, Greek yoghurt, whey protein, cocoa powder and milk to a blender or food processor. Pulse until the mixture has a smooth and creamy consistency.

2. Use a spatula to guide the mixture into a plastic container. Grate over the dark chocolate, stir well and place in the freezer for 2 hours.

3. Remove the ice cream from the freezer and stir with a spoon (this creates a light, creamy texture).

4. To serve your ice cream, remove from the freezer 10 minutes beforehand for an easy scoop (store for up to 1 month).

5. Enjoy the ice cream by itself or serve along with fruit, nuts or seeds of your choice.

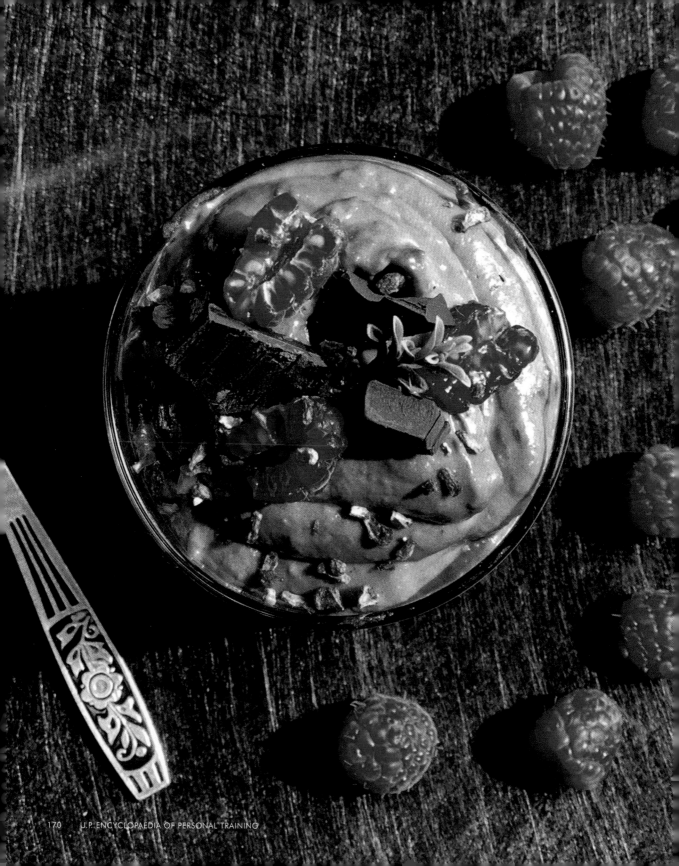

REFEED INSPIRATION

AVOCADO CHOCOLATE MOUSSE

PREP TIME: Under 10 mins.
COOL TIME: Under 30 mins.

CALORIES	PROTEIN	FAT	CARBS
235 kCal	15 g	15 g	10 g

EQUIPMENT

- Digital food scales.
- Blender or food processor.
- Spatula.
- Serving bowl.
- Grater.

INGREDIENTS

Note: makes 2 portions.

- 1/2 avocado, peeled.
- 30g chocolate whey protein.
- 1 tbsp unsweetened cacao powder.
- 1 tbsp coconut oil, melted.
- 1 tbsp 0% fat Greek yoghurt.
- 1 tsp honey.

Serve with:

- 10g 70-90% dark chocolate.
- 30g raspberries.
- Fruit, nuts and seeds of choice - see transformation food tables.

METHOD

1. Add the avocado, whey protein, cacao powder, coconut oil, Greek yoghurt and honey to a blender or food processor. Pulse until the mixture has a smooth and creamy consistency.

2. Use a spatula to guide the mixture into a serving bowl. Chill in the fridge for 15-30 minutes until the coconut oil sets in the mix creating a thicker texture.

3. Remove the mousse from the fridge, grate over the dark chocolate and serve topped with fresh raspberries and any extra fruit, nuts or seeds of your choice.

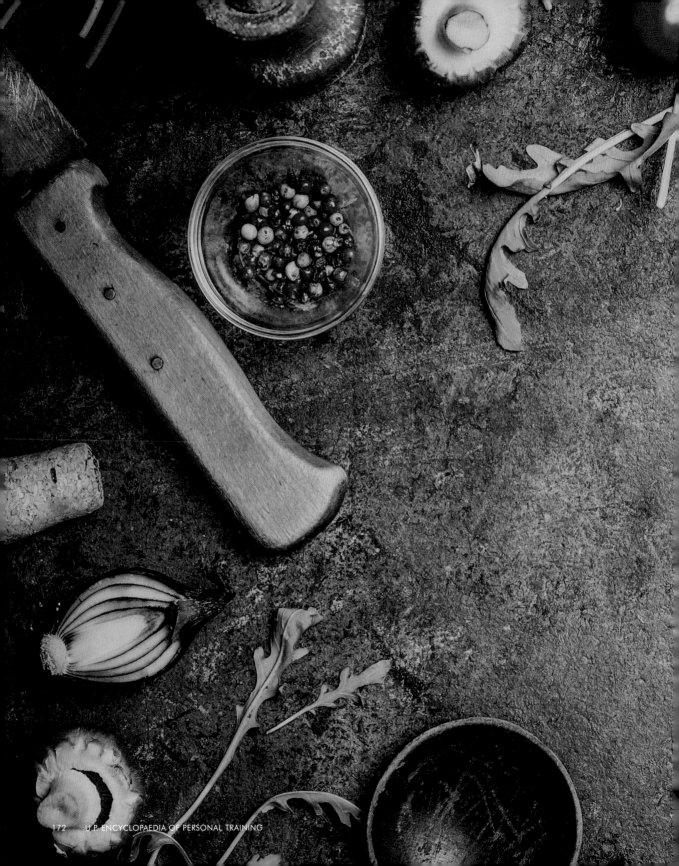

EXTRAS

Transformation Case Studies
Supplements
Quick Start Nutrition Targets
Glossary
References
About the Authors

TRANSFORMATION CASE STUDIES

MIKE

CLIENT PROFILE		BEFORE	AFTER
Bodyweight		115kg	**75kg** ▼
Body fat percentage		40%+	**15%** ▼

CLIENT PROFILE

Age: 40s
Transformation time frame: 33 weeks

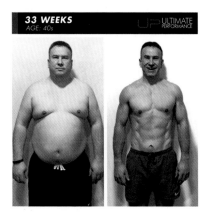
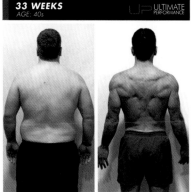
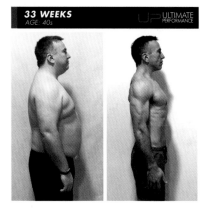

When Mike started his transformation, he weighed 115kg and his diet was out of control.

Working long hours as a construction company director meant he skipped breakfast, snacked throughout the day and relied heavily on takeaways in the evening.

"My biggest mistake before joining Ultimate Performance (U.P.) was portion control. I ate what I wanted, when I wanted".

"I previously tried a meal replacement diet (shakes and soups) and lost three stone in 12 weeks. The diet was not sustainable though and I gained the weight back, plus extra, and ended up weighing more than when I started!".

In just 33 weeks, Mike lost 40kg in bodyweight, 40 inches from his waistline and dropped from a body fat percentage of over 40% to 15%.

Completing his transformation has helped Mike go from feeling constantly tired and sluggish, to feeling energised and positive.

"I am a lot more in control of my diet now. I feel great and wake up looking forward to what each day brings. I feel 10 years younger since starting at U.P."

TRANSFORMATION HABITS	PRE-TRANSFORMATION	TRANSFORMATION
MEAL PLANNING	Too busy for breakfast. Snacked on sandwiches, crisps and chocolate bars throughout the day. Huge takeaway meals for dinner. Usual dinner out was burger and chips.	4 balanced meals spaced evenly throughout the day. Used a meal-delivery service during the day and prepared own dinner. Used digital food scales and tracked diet in MyFitnessPal (when preparing own meals). Researched restaurant menus and tried to save calories earlier in the day.
PROTEIN	100g of protein per day.	Included a protein source at every meal and aimed for 200g per day.
FRUIT AND VEGETABLES	Minimal.	A key part of every meal.
WATER	1 litre per day.	3-4 litres per day.
CAFFEINE	5-6 coffees per day (all with sugar and milk).	2 black coffees per day.
ALCOHOL	2-3 late nights out drinking per week.	No alcohol during transformation.
TRAINING	Commuted via cabs/tube and averaged 3,000 steps per day. No resistance training.	3-4 resistance training and 1-2 HIIT workouts per week. Walked to and from work and averaged at least 10,000 steps per day.

TRANSFORMATION CASE STUDIES
—
ANDY

<table>
<tr><td></td><td>**BEFORE**</td><td>**AFTER**</td></tr>
<tr><td>**Bodyweight**</td><td>115kg</td><td>89kg ▼</td></tr>
<tr><td>**Body fat percentage**</td><td>30%</td><td>10% ▼</td></tr>
</table>

CLIENT PROFILE

Age: 40s
Transformation time frame: 33 weeks

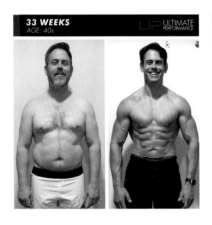
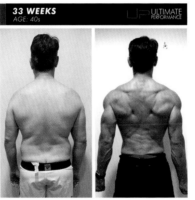
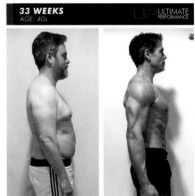

Andy's weight had been slowly increasing for 15 years before he started working with Ultimate Performance (U.P.).

He played rugby professionally when he was younger and never had to pay much attention to his diet due to the demanding training schedule.

""Back in my playing days, I could get away with eating pretty much anything I wanted. We would drink after games, eat lots of takeaways, and never put on a pound!"

But, a severe shoulder injury put a stop to his sporting career and with the transition to a more sedentary lifestyle, his weight slowly crept up.

With the help of his trainer, Andy managed to lose 26kg and cut his body fat down by two thirds in 33 weeks. He has dropped from wearing 3XL clothing to a medium, has started playing rugby again at the age of 47 and completed a photoshoot to mark the end of his transformation (alongside his wife who also transformed at U.P.).

"Looking back, 33 weeks ago I had a full beard, was not happy with myself, and would try to hide in extra clothing in photos. Now, who cares, bring it on!"

TRANSFORMATION HABITS	PRE-TRANSFORMATION	TRANSFORMATION
MEAL PLANNING	Never ate breakfast and often forgot to eat during the day at work. Frequent meals out and takeaways. Only form of portion control was whatever fitted on the plate.	4 balanced meals spaced evenly throughout the day. Batch cooked food in advance for the week. Used digital food scales and tracked diet in MyFitnessPal. Dined out regularly, but made smart choices, e.g. fillet steak and vegetables.
PROTEIN	Typical main meal was Spaghetti bolognese, which was 95% carbohydrates and a little meat in the sauce.	Included a protein source at every meal and aimed for 200g per day. Main protein sources were chicken, beef mince, salmon and prawns.
FRUIT AND VEGETABLES	'Token serving' with evening meal to make the plate look a little less white.	A key part of every meal.
WATER	Very rarely drank water by itself.	4 litres per day.
CAFFEINE	5-6 teas per day.	1 black coffee per day.
ALCOHOL	Tee-total.	No change.
TRAINING	2-3 bike rides per week but no resistance training. Sedentary lifestyle and never got close to 10,000 steps per day.	3-4 resistance training workouts per week and daily LISS workouts on exercise bike at home. Averaged at least 10,000 steps per day.

TRANSFORMATION CASE STUDIES

—

NEIL

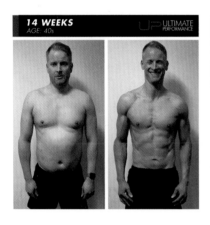
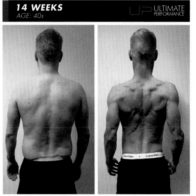
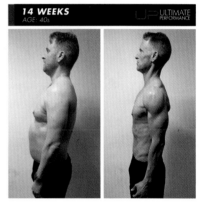

Neil was by no means new to the fitness lifestyle when he joined Ultimate Performance (U.P.).

In fact, he had spent five years going it alone in the pursuit of increased size and strength before deciding to start his transformation challenge.

However, a complete lack of dietary awareness meant that he was sabotaging all his hard work in the gym.

"Before joining U.P., I definitely managed to increase my size, but I'd say that it was mostly in the form of body fat, especially around my waist."

"I thought fat gain was an inevitable side effect of trying to build muscle, but I got a real shock when I saw my 'before' pictures."

Frustrated with his lack of results and confused by all the conflicting information in magazines and online, Neil joined U.P. and with the help of his trainer managed to lose 19kg and more than half his body fat in just 14 weeks.

"Coming to U.P. and letting them advise and make decisions on what approach to take was essential for someone like me."

"Without this structure, I'd have been completely lost and probably still in the same shape that I was three months ago."

TRANSFORMATION HABITS	PRE-TRANSFORMATION	TRANSFORMATION
MEAL PLANNING	No awareness of calories or macronutrients when deciding what to eat. Standard weekend breakfast: 3 x bacon and egg McMuffin and a hash brown. TV eater – mindlessly snacked on ice cream and chocolate bars.	Spaced meals evenly throughout the day to help combat evening cravings. Got into a meal planning routine and had go-to meals – salmon, broccoli and sweet potato was a favourite! Limited dining out but favoured steak restaurants when he did. Ordered extra vegetables and a mint tea for dessert. Used digital food scales and tracked diet in MyFitnessPal.
PROTEIN	Roughly 300g of protein per day. Used to think that the more protein you ate, the more muscle you built.	200g of protein per day.
FRUIT AND VEGETABLES	Always made an effort with vegetables, but hardly ever ate fruit.	A key part of every meal and even started looking forwards to steamed broccoli!
WATER	Less than 1 litre per day.	4 litres per day.
CAFFEINE	Several espressos per day while at work.	No caffeine during transformation. Post transformation, 1-2 black coffees per day.
ALCOHOL	Quit smoking and cut down on drinking before starting transformation.	Tee-total during transformation.
TRAINING	Resistance trained for 5 years, but had no specific goal and lacked direction. Never paid attention to step count, so no idea on pre-transformation average.	3 resistance training and 2 HIIT cardio workouts per week. Averaged at least 10,000 steps per day.

TRANSFORMATION CASE STUDIES

—

DEE

	BEFORE	AFTER
Bodyweight	60kg	49kg ▼
Body fat percentage	34%	12% ▼

CLIENT PROFILE

Age: 30s
Transformation time frame: 22 weeks

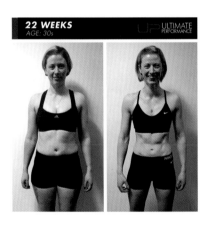
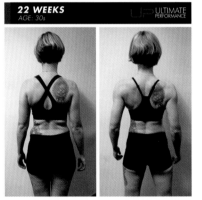
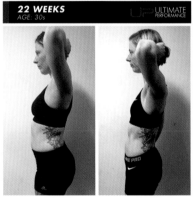

Before joining Ultimate Performance (U.P.), Dee had no idea how much her diet and lifestyle were impacting on her health and body composition.

She suffered from anxiety, psoriasis (an inflammatory skin condition) and had endured 20 years of chronic insomnia.

As a senior executive at a global company, she saw her diet as a barrier to productivity and felt that by starving herself, or eating on-the-go, she was being efficient.

"I'd never seen food as fuel before. I'd seen it as this inconvenience that I had to do in between trying to do everything else."

During her 22 week transformation, Dee lost 11kg and managed to resolve several health complaints that years of medications and treatments had failed to address.

Her psoriasis cleared up within weeks of starting and she now gets eight hours of quality sleep a night. She has also switched jobs after over 12 years with the same company, completed a photoshoot and ran a marathon.

"I'm 37 and now have measurements smaller than I did when I left university. I've knocked over 10 years off my age in terms of being physically and mentally fitter and stronger."

TRANSFORMATION HABITS	PRE-TRANSFORMATION	TRANSFORMATION
MEAL PLANNING	Never ate breakfast and rarely had lunch (apart from boozy weekend brunches). Ate dinner late at night and mostly takeaways. Only cooked at home once every few weeks. Saw eating as an inconvenience and thought skipping meals was being efficient.	4 balanced meals spaced evenly throughout the day. Scheduled meal times in diary and had easy to prepare go-to meals. Used digital food scales and tracked diet in MyFitnessPal. Planned ahead and included a weekly dinner out with partner in meal plan.
PROTEIN	'What is protein...?' Used to think that eating protein and lifting weights bulked you up.	120g of protein per day. Favourite protein-based meal was smoked salmon and poached eggs for breakfast (took less than 3 minutes to prepare at work).
FRUIT AND VEGETABLES	Ate a carbohydrate-rich diet, but very few fruit and vegetables.	A key part of every meal.
WATER	Very rarely drank water by itself.	3-4 litres per day.
CAFFEINE	12 coffee/teas per day.	1-2 black coffees per day.
ALCOHOL	14 large glasses of wine per week.	No alcohol during transformation. Post-transformation, 2-3 glasses of wine per week, but often goes a month without.
TRAINING	No resistance training. Sedentary lifestyle due to always feeling physically exhausted (caused by lack of sleep).	3-4 resistance training workouts per week. Averaged at least 10,000 steps per day. Trained for and completed marathon at the end of her transformation.

TRANSFORMATION CASE STUDIES
—
KELLY

	BEFORE	AFTER
Bodyweight	65kg	50kg ▼
Body fat percentage	40%	27% ▼

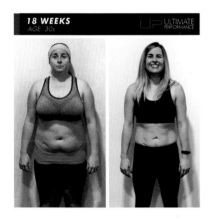
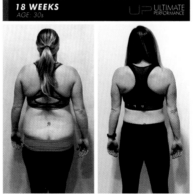
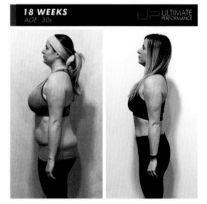

Kelly's weight had spiralled out of control before joining Ultimate Performance (U.P.).

She had gone from being fit, healthy, and competing in triathlons, to what she describes as being a 'fat lazy blob'.

The biggest challenges Kelly faced were trying to find consistency with her diet while commuting between London and Paris for work, and overcoming her emotional eating habits.

"My diet gave me zero energy and made me lethargic. I was using food and alcohol as a comfort blanket to mask how I was feeling. It was a viscous cycle that I could not break."

Kelly lost a total of 15kg during her 18 week transformation and went from wearing a dress size 14 to a size 6.

"I was confident that U.P. would help me shift some excess weight and get back into a routine, but I thought it would take 18 months. In my wildest dreams, I never imagined looking like I do after only 18 weeks".

"It's no exaggeration to say that U.P. has changed my life for the better. I'm the happiest I've ever been in myself (and the smallest!), and will never let myself slip back into my old ways."

TRANSFORMATION HABITS	PRE-TRANSFORMATION	TRANSFORMATION
MEAL PLANNING	Aimed for 3 meals but often skipped breakfast and snacked later in the day. Rarely prepared own food and relied on calorie-dense shop-bought and restaurant meals. No understanding of appropriate serving sizes or nutritional values of different foods.	4 balanced meals spaced evenly throughout the day. Cooked more at home, invested in Tupperware and learned to make better choices when dining out. Used digital food scales and tracked diet in MyFitnessPal.
PROTEIN	Bacon sandwich for breakfast, chicken baguette for lunch and steak for dinner (roughly 100g of protein).	Similar amount of protein, but from lean sources served with vegetables.
FRUIT AND VEGETABLES	Always made an effort and averaged 3-4 servings per day.	More consistent and now a key part of every meal.
WATER	Very rarely drank water by itself.	Included a drink before each meal to help control appetite.
CAFFEINE	1-2 teas per day (with sugar).	Swapped sugar for stevia and had the occasional diet soda.
ALCOHOL	1-2 bottles of wine on the weekend and 5-6 cocktails on a typical night out.	Tee-total during transformation. Post transformation, 1-2 drinks on the weekend.
TRAINING	Intimidated by the gym and avoided it at all costs. Hardly walked anywhere, used taxis to commute and sat stationary in meetings all day.	Joined a 24-hour gym and stayed in hotels with gyms to avoid missing workouts. 3-4 resistance training workouts per week. Averaged at least 10,000 steps per day.

TRANSFORMATION CASE STUDIES

—

VICKY

CLIENT PROFILE		BEFORE	AFTER
Age: 40s **Transformation time frame:** 20 weeks	**Bodyweight**	83kg	65kg ▼
	Body fat percentage	31%	11% ▼

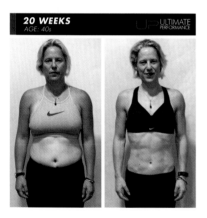
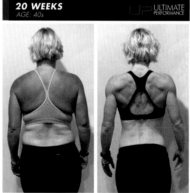
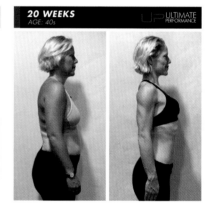

Vicky joined Ultimate Performance (U.P.) knowing she needed to make wholesale changes to her lifestyle.

As a busy chief information officer, she was working 70-hour weeks, skipping meals and drinking most nights.

"I had fallen into some really bad habits. I wasn't eating properly, I wasn't sleeping very well and I was drinking way too much."

Vicky lost 18kg over her 20 week transformation, achieved her goal of performing pull-ups with strict technique, and now has the confidence to take on physical challenges like trekking to Everest basecamp.

"It's been totally transformative. I feel like I've gotten my life back. In fact, I don't think I've ever had a body shape as good as this - even as a teenager!"

"Completing my transformation has given me the confidence to try new things. I don't hold back anymore."

TRANSFORMATION HABITS	PRE-TRANSFORMATION	TRANSFORMATION
MEAL PLANNING	Diet was not a priority. Whatever fitted around work schedule (70-hour working weeks). Skipped breakfast and often did not eat until early afternoon. Several work-related dinner and drink events per week.	4 balanced meals spaced evenly throughout the day. Batch cooked food in advance for the week. Used digital food scales and tracked diet in MyFitnessPal. Dined out regularly, but made smart choices, e.g. fillet steak and vegetables.
PROTEIN	Never thought about protein and had a maximum of 50g per day.	Included a protein source at every meal and aimed for 200g per day. Main protein sources were chicken, beef mince, salmon and prawns.
FRUIT AND VEGETABLES	1-3 servings per day, but thought 5 was impossible!	A key part of every meal.
WATER	Very rarely drank water by itself.	4 litres per day.
CAFFEINE	Depended on 3-4 coffees to survive the day.	Double espresso in the morning and fruit teas throughout the day.
ALCOHOL	2-3 glasses of wine every day and probably more on the weekends!	Tee-total during transformation. Post transformation, 1-2 drinks on the weekend.
TRAINING	No resistance training. Sedentary lifestyle and only steps were walking to the bus.	3-4 resistance training workouts per week. Cycled to and from work and averaged at least 10,000 steps per day. Trained for and completed trek to Everest base camp at the end of her transformation.

SUPPLEMENTS

THERE'S A CERTAIN DEGREE OF RELUCTANCE ON OUR PART TO EVEN INCLUDE ANYTHING IN THIS BOOK ON THE ROLE OF NUTRITIONAL SUPPLEMENTS.

Too often the supplement industry is full of outright lies about the importance of supplements in the hierarchy of needs to help you get in shape. Here's the bottom line - whilst at U.P. we are firm believers in the power of "essential" supplements that we detail in this chapter, we always advise our clients to focus their attention and budget on buying the best quality food, both for themselves and their families, long before considering using supplements.

It is true that many clients come to us with impaired digestion, and supplements can help with that because you are what you absorb (digest), not what you eat, and most modern diets have played havoc with the nutritional status of the general population. However, supplements are a tertiary consideration, lagging way behind a proper diet, exercise and stress management.

Use supplements judiciously. Do not fall into the trap of thinking they are essential. They are by their very definition "supplementary".

▶ If taking a multivitamin, you may need to reduce the doses of other supplements, e.g. magnesium.

▶ Fish oil is a combination of many different fatty acids, but the important ones are EPA and DHA. To work out the relevant amount per serving add together the values for EPA and DHA listed on the product label

▶ There are several different supplement forms of magnesium. Cheaper forms (e.g. magnesium oxide) have poor absorption rates and can cause stomach upset. We recommend and use magnesium glycinate in our magnesium supplement, 'UltraMag', for optimal absorption.

▶ Take all supplements with meals. The one exception is probiotics, which we recommend taking before meals.

SUPPLEMENT	RECOMMENDED DOSE
Multivitamin	Take daily as instructed on product label.
Fish Oil	1-2g daily.
Vitamin D3	1,000-2,000 IU daily.
Magnesium	200-400mg daily.
Digestive Enzymes	Take daily as instructed on product label.
Probiotic	Take daily as instructed on product label.

For our full range of supplements, visit our website: www.upfitness.com/shop

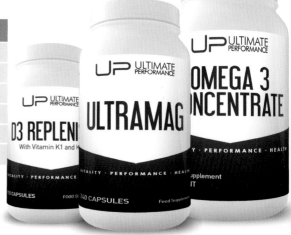

QUICK START NUTRITION TARGETS

IN THIS SECTION, WE HAVE PROVIDED *'QUICK START NUTRITION TARGETS'* YOU CAN USE TO CREATE YOUR MEAL PLAN.

To find your nutrition targets:

▶ Find the reference table that is closest to your body fat percentage estimate, e.g. if you are 17%, use the reference table for 15%.

▶ Find the bodyweight row that is closest to your bodyweight, e.g. if you weigh 67kg, use the 65kg nutrition targets.

▶ Progress to *'Transformation Foods'* to start creating your meal plan.

Note: If you weigh more than 110kg or your body fat percentage estimate is higher than 40%, use the targets for 110kg or 40% respectively.

10% BODY FAT					
BODYWEIGHT	**PROTEIN**	**FAT**	**CARBS**	**CALORIES**	**REFEED**
40kg	85	55	140	1390	1720
45kg	95	60	145	1495	1865
50kg	110	60	155	1605	2015
55kg	120	65	160	1705	2160
60kg	130	70	165	1810	2305
65kg	140	75	170	1915	2450
70kg	150	80	175	2020	2595
75kg	160	80	190	2120	2740
80kg	175	85	190	2230	2890
85kg	185	90	195	2335	3035
90kg	195	95	200	2440	3180
95kg	205	100	205	2540	3325
100kg	215	105	210	2645	3470
105kg	225	105	225	2750	3615
110kg	240	110	230	2860	3765

15% BODY FAT

BODYWEIGHT	PROTEIN	FAT	CARBS	CALORIES	REFEED
40kg	80	50	140	1325	1655
45kg	90	55	145	1425	1795
50kg	100	60	145	1520	1930
55kg	110	65	150	1615	2070
60kg	120	65	160	1710	2205
65kg	135	70	160	1810	2345
70kg	145	75	165	1910	2485
75kg	155	80	165	2000	2620
80kg	165	80	180	2100	2760
85kg	175	85	185	2195	2895
90kg	185	90	185	2295	3035
95kg	195	95	190	2385	3170
100kg	205	95	205	2485	3310
105kg	215	100	205	2580	3445
110kg	225	105	210	2680	3585

20% BODY FAT

BODYWEIGHT	PROTEIN	FAT	CARBS	CALORIES	REFEED
40kg	75	50	130	1260	1590
45kg	85	55	130	1350	1720
50kg	95	55	140	1440	1850
55kg	105	60	140	1525	1980
60kg	115	65	145	1615	2110
65kg	125	65	155	1705	2240
70kg	135	70	155	1795	2370
75kg	145	75	155	1880	2500
80kg	155	75	170	1970	2630
85kg	165	80	170	2060	2760
90kg	175	85	170	2150	2890
95kg	180	85	185	2230	3015
100kg	190	90	190	2320	3145
105kg	200	95	190	2410	3275
110kg	210	95	200	2500	3405

25% BODY FAT

BODYWEIGHT	PROTEIN	FAT	CARBS	CALORIES	REFEED
40kg	70	45	130	1195	1525
45kg	80	50	130	1280	1650
50kg	90	55	125	1360	1770
55kg	100	55	135	1435	1890
60kg	110	60	135	1520	2015
65kg	115	60	150	1600	2135
70kg	125	65	150	1680	2255
75kg	135	70	150	1760	2380
80kg	145	70	160	1840	2500
85kg	155	75	155	1920	2620
90kg	160	80	160	2000	2740
95kg	170	80	170	2080	2865
100kg	180	85	170	2160	2985
105kg	190	85	180	2240	3105
110kg	200	90	180	2325	3230

30% BODY FAT

BODYWEIGHT	PROTEIN	FAT	CARBS	CALORIES	REFEED
40kg	65	45	115	1130	1460
45kg	75	45	125	1205	1575
50kg	85	50	125	1280	1690
55kg	90	50	135	1345	1800
60kg	100	55	130	1420	1915
65kg	110	60	130	1495	2030
70kg	120	60	140	1570	2145
75kg	125	65	140	1635	2255
80kg	135	65	145	1710	2370
85kg	145	70	145	1785	2485
90kg	150	70	155	1855	2595
95kg	160	75	155	1925	2710
100kg	170	80	150	2000	2825
105kg	175	80	165	2070	2935
110kg	185	85	160	2145	3050

35% BODY FAT

BODYWEIGHT	PROTEIN	FAT	CARBS	CALORIES	REFEED
40kg	60	40	115	1065	1395
45kg	70	45	115	1135	1505
50kg	80	45	120	1200	1610
55kg	85	50	120	1260	1715
60kg	95	50	125	1325	1820
65kg	100	55	125	1390	1925
70kg	110	55	130	1455	2030
75kg	115	60	130	1515	2135
80kg	125	60	135	1580	2240
85kg	135	65	130	1645	2345
90kg	140	65	140	1710	2450
95kg	150	70	135	1770	2555
100kg	155	70	145	1835	2660
105kg	165	75	140	1900	2765
110kg	170	75	155	1965	2870

40% BODY FAT

BODYWEIGHT	PROTEIN	FAT	CARBS	CALORIES	REFEED
40kg	60	40	100	1005	1335
45kg	65	40	110	1060	1430
50kg	70	45	110	1115	1525
55kg	80	45	110	1170	1625
60kg	85	50	110	1225	1720
65kg	95	50	115	1285	1820
70kg	100	50	125	1340	1915
75kg	110	55	115	1395	2015
80kg	115	55	125	1450	2110
85kg	120	60	120	1505	2205
90kg	130	60	125	1565	2305
95kg	135	65	125	1615	2400
100kg	145	65	130	1675	2500
105kg	150	65	135	1730	2595
110kg	160	70	130	1790	2695

GLOSSARY

3,500kcal Rule

A meal planning guideline based on the fact that a pound (0.45kg) of body fat contains 3,500kcal.

Activity Energy Expenditure (AEE)

The number of calories you burn during purposeful exercise (resistance training and formal cardio) and all other physical activity that is not sleeping or eating.

Activity Multiplier

A method of expressing how active you are each day as a number. For example, if your RMR is 2,000kcal and you expend an additional 1,000kcal through activity, your multiplier would be 'x 1.5' (3,000/2,000). Most people fall somewhere between 1.4 and 2.2.

Adherence

A measure of how closely you follow the nutrition and training guidelines that make up your transformation program.

Body Fat Percentage (%)

The weight of all the fat on your body (fat mass) divided by your total bodyweight and expressed as a percentage.

Calorie Balance (also known as 'Energy Balance')

The relationship between the energy (measured in calories) that enters your body from food and drink and exits as part of your total daily energy expenditure (TDEE). Your body's calorie balance can be positive, negative or neutral.

Calorie Density

The number of calories provided per unit measure of food. Foods that contain a high number of calories per serving are 'calorie-dense', whereas the opposite applies for 'calorie-sparse' foods.

Calorie Shifting

A meal planning tactic that you can use to increase your calorie allowance on a specific day by taking calories from another day in the week. Calorie shifting results in an uneven calorie distribution across the week that is also known as 'calorie cycling'.

Calories

A unit of measurement, like how metres are a unit of length and kilograms are a unit of mass. In the context of diet and exercise, we typically use calories to measure: (1) the amount of energy provided by food and drink, (2) the amount of energy you expend, or 'burn', each day through physical activity.

Essential Nutrient

A nutrient that you require for normal physiological functioning but that your body cannot create on its own. As a result, you must obtain it from a dietary source.

Formal Cardio

Structured cardio workouts deliberately performed as part of your training program.

Guesstimate

An estimate of the nutritional value (calorie and macronutrient content) of a meal based on a combination of guesswork and research.

Hidden Calories

An ingredient that adds to the calorie count of a meal but is not immediately apparent if you are not preparing the meal yourself. For example, oil and butter added by chefs to restaurant meals.

High-Intensity Interval Training (HIIT)

A type of formal cardio that alternates short periods of high-intensity exercise (RPE 7-10) with less intense recovery periods (RPE 2-3), e.g. sprint intervals.

Lean Body Mass (LBM)

A component of body composition, which you can calculate by subtracting your fat mass from your total bodyweight.

Low-Intensity Steady State (LISS) Cardio

A type of formal cardio that involves performing a low-intensity activity (RPE 1-4) for extended periods of time, e.g. treadmill walking.

Macronutrients

A type of nutrient that your body requires in large amounts. There are three macronutrients (protein, fat and carbohydrate), which all provide your body with a certain amount of energy in addition to performing several other important roles.

Maintenance Calorie Intake

The number of calories you need to consume to maintain your current bodyweight.

Meal Plan

An action plan for how to approach your diet for a specific period, typically one week.

Measurement Error

The difference between a measured quantity and its actual value.

Metabolic Adaptations

Adaptations made by your body in response to sustained caloric restriction to slow down the rate of fat loss and conserve energy. For example, reduced energy expenditure from NEAT, changes in hormone levels and increased cravings and food-focused behaviour.

Moderate-Intensity Steady State (MISS) Cardio

A type of formal cardio that involves performing a moderate-intensity activity (RPE 5-6) for extended periods of time, e.g. 5km run.

Non-Exercise Activity Thermogenesis (NEAT)

The number of calories you burn performing all physical activity that is not purposeful exercise, sleeping or eating. NEAT consists of a voluntary component, e.g. walking, and an involuntary component that is beyond your conscious control, e.g. fidgeting.

Refeed

A planned period of increased calorie intake while dieting that can last anywhere from a few hours up to a few days.

Resistance Training

A type of exercise that forces your muscles to work against resistance provided by your own bodyweight, free weights (dumbbells and barbells) and machines.

Resting Metabolic Rate (RMR)

The minimum amount of energy your body needs to maintain vital life functions at rest, such as your heart rate and breathing.

RMR is often used interchangeably with the term, 'basal metabolic rate' (BMR), which refers to the same concept, but there is a technical difference in how you measure them.

Thermic Effect of Food (TEF)

The number of calories you burn digesting, absorbing and processing foods for use and storage inside your body.

Total Daily Energy Expenditure (TDEE)

The total number of calories you burn each day. TDEE is the total of all calories burned via RMR, AEE and TEF.

REFERENCES

SETTING UP FOR SUCCESS

Areta, J., Burke, L., Camera, D., West, D., Crawshay, S., Moore, D., Stellingwerff, T., Phillips, S., Hawley, J. and Coffey, V. (2014). Reduced resting skeletal muscle protein synthesis is rescued by resistance exercise and protein ingestion following short-term energy deficit. American Journal of Physiology-Endocrinology and Metabolism, 306(8), pp.E989-E997.

Helms, E., Fitschen, P., Aragon, A., Cronin, J. and Schoenfeld, B. (2015). Recommendations for natural bodybuilding contest preparation: resistance and cardiovascular training. The Journal of Sports Medicine and Physical Fitness, 55(3), pp.164-178.

Helms, E., Morgan, A. and Valdez, A. (2015). The Muscle and Strength Pyramid: Nutrition. muscleandstrengthpyramids.com, pp.29-59.

Loeffelholz, C. (2018). The Role of Non-exercise Activity Thermogenesis in Human Obesity. [online] Ncbi.nlm.nih.gov. Available at: https://www.ncbi.nlm.nih.gov/books/NBK279077/ [Accessed 2 Jul. 2018].

Levine, J., Vander Weg, M., Hill, J. and Klesges, R. (2006). Non-Exercise Activity Thermogenesis: The Crouching Tiger Hidden Dragon of Societal Weight Gain. Arteriosclerosis, Thrombosis, and Vascular Biology, 26(4), pp.729-736.

Levine, J. (2007). Nonexercise activity thermogenesis - liberating the life-force. Journal of Internal Medicine, 262(3), pp.273-287.

Longland, T., Oikawa, S., Mitchell, C., Devries, M. and Phillips, S. (2016). Higher compared with lower dietary protein during an energy deficit combined with intense exercise promotes greater lean mass gain and fat mass loss: a randomized trial. The American Journal of Clinical Nutrition, 103(3), pp.738-746.

Nader, G. (2006). Concurrent Strength and Endurance Training: From Molecules to Man. Medicine & Science in Sports & Exercise, 38(11), pp.1965-1970.

Wilson, J., Marin, P., Rhea, M., Wilson, S., Loenneke, J. and Anderson, J. (2012). Concurrent Training: A meta- analysis examining interference of aerobic and resistance exercises. Journal of Strength and Conditioning Research, 26(8), pp.2293-2307.

TRANSFORMATION NUMBERS

Fao.org. (2018). Human energy requirements. [online] Available at: http://www.fao.org/docrep/007/y5686e/y5686e00.htm [Accessed 2 Jul. 2018].

Gardner, C., Trepanowski, J., Del Gobbo, L., Hauser, M., Rigdon, J., Ioannidis, J., Desai, M. and King, A. (2018). Effect of Low-Fat vs Low-Carbohydrate Diet on 12-Month Weight Loss in Overweight Adults and the Association With Genotype Pattern or Insulin Secretion. JAMA, 319(7), pp.667-669.

Garthe, I., Raastad, T., Refsnes, P., Koivisto, A. and Sundgot-Borgen, J. (2011). Effect of Two Different Weight-Loss Rates on Body Composition and Strength and Power-Related Performance in Elite Athletes. International Journal of Sport Nutrition and Exercise Metabolism, 21(2), pp.97-104.

Hall, K. (2007). What is the required energy deficit per unit weight loss?. International Journal of Obesity, 32(3), pp.573-576.

Helms, E., Aragon, A. and Fitschen, P. (2014). Evidence-based recommendations for natural bodybuilding contest preparation: nutrition and supplementation. Journal of the International Society of Sports Nutrition, 11(1), p.1-20.

Helms, E., Morgan, A. and Valdez, A. (2015). The Muscle and Strength Pyramid: Nutrition. muscleandstrengthpyramids.com, pp.26-80.

Jäger, R., Kerksick, C., Campbell, B., Cribb, P., Wells, S., Skwiat, T., Purpura, M., Ziegenfuss, T., Ferrando, A., Arent, S., Smith-Ryan, A., Stout, J., Arciero, P., Ormsbee, M., Taylor, L., Wilborn, C., Kalman, D., Kreider, R., Willoughby, D., Hoffman, J., Krzykowski, J. and Antonio, J. (2017). International Society of Sports Nutrition Position Stand: protein and exercise. Journal of the International Society of Sports Nutrition, 14(1), pp.1-25.

Katch, F., Katch, V., McArdle, W. (2014). 'Exercise Physiology: nutrition, energy, and Human Performance', 8th ed., Lippincott Williams and Wilkins, pp.8-38.

McDonald, L. (2017). The Women's Book: Volume 1. A Guide to Nutrition, Fat Loss, and Muscle Gain. 1st ed. Austin, TX, Lyle McDonald Publishing, pp.157-185.

Thomas, D., Martin, C., Lettieri, S., Bredlau, C., Kaiser, K., Church, T., Bouchard, C. and Heymsfield, S. (2013). Can a weight loss of one pound a week be achieved with a 3500-kcal deficit? Commentary on a commonly accepted rule. International Journal of Obesity, 37(12), pp.1611-1613.

TRANSFORMATION FOODS

Institute of Medicine. 2005. Dietary Reference Intakes for Energy, Carbohydrate, Fiber, Fat, Fatty Acids, Cholesterol, Protein, and Amino Acids. Washington, DC: The National Academies Press, pp. 265-768.

Katch, F., Katch, V., McArdle, W. (2014). 'Exercise Physiology: nutrition, energy, and Human Performance', 8th ed., Lippincott Williams and Wilkins, pp.8-38.

McDonald, L. (2017). The Women's Book: Volume 1. A Guide to Nutrition, Fat Loss, and Muscle Gain. 1st ed. Austin, TX, Lyle McDonald Publishing, pp.199-218.

Scientific Opinion on the safety of caffeine. (2015). EFSA Journal, 13(5), pp.1-74.

U.S. Food and Drug Administration. (2018). Additional Information about High-Intensity Sweeteners Permitted for Use in Food in the United States. [online] Available at: https://www.fda.gov/Food/IngredientsPackagingLabeling/FoodAdditivesIngredients/ucm397725.htm#Aspartame [Accessed 2 Jul. 2018].

REFERENCES

TRANSFORMATION MEAL PLANNING

Kerksick, C., Arent, S., Schoenfeld, B., Stout, J., Campbell, B., Wilborn, C., Taylor, L., Kalman, D., Smith-Ryan, A., Kreider, R., Willoughby, D., Arciero, P., VanDusseldorp, T., Ormsbee, M., Wildman, R., Greenwood, M., Ziegenfuss, T., Aragon, A. and Antonio, J. (2017). International society of sports nutrition position stand: nutrient timing. Journal of the International Society of Sports Nutrition, 14(1), pp.1-21.

La Bounty, P., Campbell, B., Wilson, J., Galvan, E., Berardi, J., Kleiner, S., Kreider, R., Stout, J., Ziegenfuss, T., Spano, M., Smith, A. and Antonio, J. (2011). International Society of Sports Nutrition position stand: meal frequency. Journal of the International Society of Sports Nutrition, 8(1), pp.1-12.

Phillips, S., Tipton, K., Aarsland, A., Wolf, S. and Wolfe, R. (1997). Mixed muscle protein synthesis and breakdown after resistance exercise in humans. American Journal of Physiology-Endocrinology and Metabolism, 273(1), pp.E99-E107.

Schoenfeld, B., Aragon, A. and Krieger, J. (2015). Effects of meal frequency on weight loss and body composition: a meta-analysis. Nutrition Reviews, 73(2), pp.69-82.

Trexler, E., Smith-Ryan, A. and Norton, L. (2014). Metabolic adaptation to weight loss: implications for the athlete. Journal of the International Society of Sports Nutrition, 11(1), pp.1-7.

PROGRESS ASSESSMENT AND HOW TO MAKE CHANGES

Aragon, A. (2014). What causes weight loss plateaus, and how can they be overcome?. Alan Aragon's Research Review, pp.17-18.

Hume, P. and Marfell-Jones, M. (2008). The importance of accurate site location for skinfold measurement. Journal of Sports Sciences, 26(12), pp.1333-1340.

Katch, F., Katch, V., McArdle, W. (2014). 'Exercise Physiology: nutrition, energy, and Human Performance', 8th ed., Lippincott Williams and Wilkins, pp.731-763.

Stewart, A., Marfell-Jones, M., Olds, T. and Hans De Ridder, J. (2011). International Standards for Anthropometric Assessment. 1st ed. International Society for the Advancement of Kinanthropometry, pp.1-76.

ABOUT
THE
AUTHORS

ABOUT THE AUTHORS

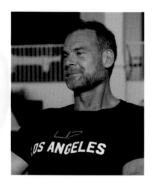

NICK MITCHELL

Global CEO and Founder,
Ultimate Performance

Nick Mitchell is the founder of Ultimate Performance - the only global personal training business in the world, operating their own gyms across four different continents.

Hailed as 'one of the world's leading body composition experts' by multiple high profile publications, Nick is renowned for developing methodologies that have helped hundreds of thousands of people get in the best shape of their lives in the quickest possible time.

A multiple best-selling book author and a columnist in everything from Muscle & Fitness, Men's Health, Men's Fitness, and Flex, to the UK's Daily Telegraph, Nick spends what little spare time he has trying and failing to teach his children that daddy knows best.

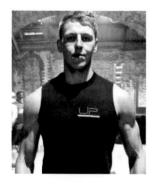

JONATHAN TAYLOR

Deputy Head of Education
at Ultimate Performance

Body Transformation Meal Plan Design is the second book that Jonathan Taylor has co-written alongside Nick Mitchell.

Jonathan is the Deputy Head of Education at Ultimate Performance (U.P.) and is an instrumental part of the team that continues to cement U.P.'s place at the top of the results-producing tree across the global personal training industry.

A huge proponent of the benefits of hard work, Jonathan doesn't waste his time on social media but you can see multiple examples of his work on the U.P. Twitter (@upfitness) and Instagram pages (@upfitnesslive).

ACKNOWLEDGEMENTS

FROM NICK MITCHELL

The blood, sweat and tears of this book all belong to Jonathan Taylor. I do the easy bit and then he does all the real work. If you've derived the results that I know you can get if you follow the plan, then the lion's share of the credit rests with him.

As always though, no book is a solo project. Praise and thanks have to go to Andrew Cheung, U.P.'s Head of Graphic Design, who built the pages that you've just read, as well as to the entire U.P. team who have worked so tirelessly for the last decade to help us refine our processes so that we're unquestionably the world's number one results-producing personal training team.

FROM JONATHAN TAYLOR

Once again, I would like to take this opportunity to officially thank Nick Mitchell for the impact he has had on my career to date.

Working on the first two instalments of the U.P. encyclopaedia series together has been a life-changing experience and one that I will never forget.

I also owe another huge thanks to my parents, Michael and Linda Taylor. After helping me to research and proof-read this book for several months, I am now confident that they know more about resistance training and nutrition than the average personal trainer!

Finally, I also owe huge thanks to Andrew Cheung for bringing this book to life, to Sean Murphy for his ongoing friendship and mentorship, and to all my clients past and present who I continue to learn from every day.